3-31-76

The Child with Convulsions

A Guide for Parents, Teachers,
Counselors, and Medical Personnel

A Guide for Parents, Teachers, Counselors, and Medical Personnel

The Child
with Convulsions

HENRY W. BAIRD, M.D.

Professor of Pediatrics,
Temple University School of Medicine,
and Pediatric Neurologist,
St. Christopher's Hospital for Children,
Philadelphia, Pennsylvania

GRUNE & STRATTON

A Subsidiary of Harcourt Brace Jovanovich, Publishers

New York   San Francisco   London

Library of Congress Cataloging in Publication Data
Baird, Henry W.
    The child with convulsions.
    Bibliography: p.
    1. Convulsions. 2. Children—Diseases. I. Title.
RJ496.C7B35   618.9′28′45   72–1870
ISBN 0–8089–0757–3

Grune & Stratton, Inc.
111 Fifth Avenue
New York, New York 10003

Library of Congress Catalog Card Number 72–1870
International Standard Book Number 0–8089–0757–3
Printed in the United States of America

CONTENTS

FOREWORD *by W. E. Nelson, M.D.*   vii

PREFACE   ix

PART ONE: *The Diagnosis*   1

AN INTRODUCTION   3
   Types of seizures and their causes   6
   The general course of diagnosis and treatment   8
THE CONSULTATION   11
DIAGNOSTIC PROCEDURES   16
   Psychological testing   16
   Psychological tests which may be helpful   21
   Psychological report   28
   The electroencephalogram   30

PART TWO: *Convulsions and Their
             Treatment*   43

"FITS" AND FAINTS   45
   Types of seizures   45
CONDITIONS RESEMBLING SEIZURES   55
   Conditions of uncertain nature   56
   Nonconvulsive conditions   57
MEDICAL TREATMENT OF SEIZURES   62
   Drugs   63
   Non-drug control   68

CONDITIONS WHICH MAY BE ASSOCIATED
WITH CONVULSIONS   69
    Cerebral palsy   70
    Mental retardation   71
    Other problems   74
    Body chemistry disturbances   78

PART THREE: *The Environment*   83

YOUR CHILD'S WORLD   85
    The parents' role   86
    Sports   88
    The child's relationship to his world   90
    The teen years   94
    Education   97
    Future planning   107

Appendix 1: Classification of Convulsive Disorders
            by Cause   119
Appendix 2: Origin of Brain Waves and the
            Chemical Mechanism of Seizures   121
Appendix 3: Epilepsy and Driving   122
Appendix 4: Summary of Driver's License Laws   123
Appendix 5: Glossary   130
Appendix 6: Useful References   135

INDEX   137

FOREWORD

History may record, as one of the distinct advances in the delivery of health care during the past half-century, the transfer of the day-to-day care of the person with a persistent or chronic disorder to the patient himself and to his family. The desired potential of such personal responsibility is clearly that the patient may more nearly lead an active, normal, productive, and satisfactory life. When the patient is an infant or child, the potential for success is great—provided the family, school personnel, neighbors, and, not the least, the physician understand and set such a goal as the primary objective in the management of the child.

There is a variety, actually an increasing number, of persistent disorders to be so managed. Perhaps none is a better example than epilepsy in all its clinical varieties. Many children with convulsive disorders are now leading normally active lives at home and at school, with the assurance that they can look ahead to responsible adult lives. To be sure, the outlook is not equally good for all children subject to seizures or fits; some have other handicaps: mental retardation, learning disabilities, and physical crippling, as examples. But such is also the case for many children who do not have a convulsive disorder, and significant advances have and are being made in the care and management of these children.

Basic to the adequate management of the child with a persistent disorder is an understanding of its nature and of its treatment. A broad concept by physician, family, and school teachers in particular is obviously the first step—but the critical step is the precise appraisal of the child and his environment to the end that his program can be tailored to his particular pattern and requirements.

This book is designed to provide a basis or background for such understanding. Primarily, it is for the parents of the affected child—but also it is for all those who collectively make up the child's environmental participants: the school teacher, the public health nurse, the psychologist, the child's physician, and even relatives, friends, and neighbors.

Certainly it is not Dr. Baird's intent that the parents of the child with a convulsive disorder will know or fully understand all the details contained in this comprehensive account, but it does provide three distinct advantages: 1. an opportunity for an overall understanding of the steps in diagnostic evaluation and in the immediate and long-range planning, 2. a source of reference for parents in which to check the reasons for a particular diagnostic test or therapeutic maneuver (parents do not always fully comprehend or even "hear" all of even the best attempts at explanation), and 3. perhaps most important, continuing support in their intent to live "with the disorder" and not "for it."

What Dr. Baird has done here so effectively is to share with the many families who have a child with a convulsive disorder and with their physicians what he has provided personally in his daily work at St. Christopher's Hospital for Children for his own patients and their families, as well as for the medical students and resident physicians in training. One of my privileges has been the opportunity to see at first hand and appreciate the favorable effects on patient, family, and student when the therapy of the child with a convulsive disorder not only is planned to fit his particular growth and development, but is translated into understandable language for parent and child.

When used appropriately in conjunction with continuous supportive medical guidance, this book can help materially to dispel the stigma of epilepsy and assist many an affected child and his family to achieve the basic goal—the opportunity to lead a full and satisfactory life.

Waldo E. Nelson, M.D.
Professor of Pediatrics
Temple University
School of Medicine

PREFACE

After a child has had a convulsion and the immediate problems have been solved, his parents may still have many unanswered questions. Some of these relate directly to their own child and can be answered only by a physician. Frequently, however, they are seeking more general information and want to know more about all kinds of seizures, their courses and their outcome. Written explanations directed to adults who have seizures may be merely confusing because these explanations often do not apply to children. Parents also find it difficult to understand information in medical journals and texts written for physicians.

They, and others who must cope with seizures in an individual child, will gain a good perspective on their own problem if they have a clear understanding about the possible causes, characteristics, and treatment of convulsions in general. This book is not designed to instruct them in the professional care of convulsive disorders. It is rather a guide for parents, educators, nurses, social workers, and therapists who want the child with convulsions to make the best possible adjustment to his world.

The information set out in this book is divided into the three general categories of diagnosis, treatment, and the environment in which the child lives. Because many hours of a child's life are spent at school, almost every "normal" child will eventually have some kind of difficulty there. If he happens to have had one or more seizures in the past, or received medication, it is almost certain that either of these facts will be considered the cause of his problem. Although "normal" children may have identical problems, the child with convulsions is singled out, and the presence of a chronic condition distorts the perspective of those involved in his education. Therefore, considerable space has been devoted to questions of psychological tests, proper school placement, and learning disabilities. A history of convulsions may also have a direct bearing on problems of adolescence such as driving, college, and career choice. These subjects are included briefly.

The appendices present some technical information on the causes and classification of seizures which is outside the general scope of the text but which might be interesting and useful to someone with a scientific background. A summary of the driving license regulations in each state is also presented. Some useful reading material is also listed.

To increase the usefulness of this book to those whose primary concern is with a specific area or problem, I have used cross-references liberally. The numbers appearing in brackets in the text refer not to pages but to the applicable *section numbers*.

Naturally this book reflects my point of view. I am a pediatrician who sees children referred to me by other physicians and who regards himself as one of many. Our purpose is to work together to help each child realize his highest potential.

H.W.B.

ACKNOWLEDGMENT

Many individuals, young and old, have contributed their experience, time, and energy so that this book might be completed. My colleagues know how dependent I am upon them. My special thanks are to Drs. E. C. Gordon, E. A. Spiegel and Herman Yannet, who in many ways made this book possible.

PART ONE

The Diagnosis

AN INTRODUCTION

Jane, an attractive thirteen-year-old girl, had a sudden "fainting spell" after a swimming meet at summer camp. She complained of feeling light-headed; she turned pale and suddenly lost consciousness. There were shaking movements of her arms and legs, and she foamed at the mouth. Jane woke up several minutes later complaining of a severe headache. After a sound sleep in the camp infirmary she felt entirely well. 1
What is a
convulsion?

The parents of Elaine, a bright nine-year-old, had been troubled by her lack of attention in school. She had previously been an excellent student and was making steady progress with her piano lessons. One day while her mother was washing dishes in the kitchen, she overheard Elaine practicing for a school recital. Every few minutes she skipped a note, even though she had played the piece flawlessly many times before. Her mother watched her and noticed that she seemed "out of contact" for a second or two. Elaine had no idea that she had missed any notes.

Another mother told her pediatrician that her eight-month-old son, Edward, seemed to have some difficulty in sitting up. She noticed that frequently his head dropped and at the same time both his arms jerked upward.

Charles, aged four years, suddenly began to have a peculiar habit of holding one arm out and slowly turning around in a circle and dropping to the floor. He seemed confused afterward and often did not know whether it was morning or afternoon.

Louise, two years old, was a little fussy one morning. She vomited her lunch. After she fell asleep that night, her

3

mother heard a peculiar shrill cry and found her pale and unconscious. Louise began to jerk her arms and legs rhythmically. After a minute she regained consciousness, but she felt very warm. Her temperature was 104°. The following day she broke out in a rash. She remained entirely well after the rash disappeared.

Each of these children had had a convulsion. Convulsions are also known as "seizures," "spells," or "fits." Jane had had a typical grand mal seizure of the idiopathic type (one for which no cause can be found). [See section 64.] Elaine had developed petit mal or simple staring spells [67]. Edward had had "infantile myoclonic seizures" or "lightning major" attacks [69]. Charles was having psychomotor seizures [68] and Louise had had a typical febrile convulsion, that is, one associated with the fever of a routine childhood illness [65].

The appearance of the symptoms of a convulsion of any type can be very alarming to most parents. They ask, "What is going on inside my child to show up in this frightening way?"

A seizure may be defined as a loss or alteration of consciousness associated with involuntary muscle movement (or sudden cessation of movement) and bursts of electrical activity within the brain. There is a great deal of disagreement about the basic mechanism responsible for the involuntary muscle movements and the distortion of electrical activity. It is known that each living cell in the central nervous system has a tiny electrical discharge which can be recorded. Before and during a convulsion the electrical discharges increase in frequency and strength. It is my opinion that how long the seizure lasts and what kind of symptoms occur depend upon the site of origin within the brain, the kinds of electrical discharges, and the number of cells involved. During an episode in which there is an alteration of consciousness, measurement of the small electrical discharges will almost always show whether or not the cause is within the brain and can therefore be considered a convulsive disorder. The instrument used to measure and record the electrical discharge is called an electroencephalograph (EEG) [43–53].

This explanation may clarify *what* is actually going on in the child's brain during a seizure, but it does not explain *why* there is an electrical distortion. Many attempts have been made to describe the causes of seizures in terms that are readily understood. In order to answer the question appropriately it is important to know why the question was asked at that particular time. Is the questioner worried about hereditary transmission of seizures? Is he concerned about the possible effects of seizures on intelligence or personality? Is he worried about how long treatment will be needed? Does he want to know if there is a permanent cure? Until all causes for seizures are understood no single explanation can be completely satisfactory. Nevertheless, based upon past experience, an explanation which meets the needs of that individual at that point in time can usually be found. Some of the explanations are detailed further in the appendix.

A child often has difficulty telling how he feels, so that his description of his own reaction during a seizure may be confusing to an adult. This may be particularly true to those of us who have not had a seizure. Fortunately, great writers like Dostoevski have described not only seizures but also their own reactions to them. In some instances the experience may be unique and have a vague quality which makes it impossible for the individual involved to describe them to someone else. This is particularly true for psychomotor or temporal lobe seizures [68].

**2
What does
it feel like
to have
a seizure?**

Experience during a seizure may vary from a subtle alteration of consciousness to complete unconsciousness. The seizure may be superimposed upon sleep, which is a natural fluctuation of consciousness. The awareness of one's self may change. The individual feels that he is not there, that part of his body has changed size, or that he is having a vision. A perceptual experience may occur in which sound or sight may appear to be closer or farther away than it actually is. The individual may see pictures before him, like those of a cartoon strip or on a television screen, which he can distinguish from himself. Time may be distorted, so that the experience seems to be occurring either very slowly or too fast. He may be aware that everything he is seeing has been seen before in an absolutely identical manner (dé jà vu) or, conversely, that the experience is one in which everything is being seen for the first time and is incomprehensible (jamais vu). Mood changes may occur. These include fear, depression, pleasure, displeasure, and anger. Thought and speech disorders are common. A person experiencing a seizure may repeat the same rambling tale over and over again and sound like a record that is stuck in a groove. Afterwards, he may be oblivious to the whole experience. A seizure-induced behavior disturbance during which the person might be sexually aggressive, set fires, or commit other antisocial acts in a dream-like state is extremely rare. *I have never seen a child whose behavior could be so explained.* In those instances that this explantion is suggested, there are usually other evidences of a severe, pre-existing behavior disorder.

TYPES OF SEIZURES AND THEIR CAUSES

3 General classification of seizures Seizures can be classified as *acute* (or *nonrecurrent*) and *recurrent*. Acute, in this sense, means sudden and single rather than chronic and repetitive. It has nothing to do with the severity of the convulsion. The term epilepsy (from the Greek epilepsia: seizure) merely means a recurring convulsive disorder. If a cause cannot be found, the term *idiopathic* or *cryptogenic* epilepsy is appropriate. If a brain abnormality has been found to be the cause of the recurrent spells, *organic* or *symptomatic* epilepsy is said to be present. The physician can often predict which child will have recurrent seizures if he finds the cause of the first convulsion. A detailed technical classification of epileptic seizures currently in use is given in Appendix 1.

4 Causes of acute (non-recurrent) seizures Underlying causes of acute or nonrecurrent seizures are extremely varied. The convusion is merely a symptom of another disease which has somehow triggered the cells of the brain to produce an irregular electrical discharge. Some causes of acute seizures may be listed here:

a. Fever, accompanying a routine illness in a child under six

b. Infections (for example, meningitis [or infection of the tissues covering the brain], encephalitis [or infection of the brain itself], brain abscess, tetanus, malaria, dysentery)

c. Brain hemorrhage from birth injury or other injury or from blood disorders such as hemophilia or sickle cell disease

d. Poisons, such as lead and camphor

e. Sudden lack of oxygen, as in near-drowning

f. Sudden swelling of the brain as a result of water retention as in kidney disease

g. Brain tumor

A more detailed technical list will be found in Appendix 1.

Recurrent convulsions for which no cause can be found are called idiopathic seizures. Most recurrent convulsions fall into this category. There are also some specific causes for recurrent seizures. Some are easily recognized, but, in many instances, clinical observation for several years may be necessary to arrive at a firm diagnosis. Some of the more common causes are listed here:

5 Causes of recurrent seizures

a. Permanent damage to the brain following hemorrhage from birth injury or accidental injury

b. Permanent damage following infectious disease, lack of oxygen, or poisons

c. Degeneration of brain tissue caused by chronic disease of the central nervous system

d. Congenital malformations of the brain

e. Parasitic brain infections such as syphilis

f. Chronic disorders of body chemistry, for example, low blood sugar, abnormal calcium metabolism, untreated phenylketonuria

g. Kidney failure

A more complete technical list of causes of recurrent seizures may be found in Appendix 1.

During the first two years of life convulsions from any cause are more common than at any other period. The most frequent causes of seizures in very young infants are birth injuries affecting the brain, including the effects of oxygen lack, of bleeding, and congenital malformations of the brain. Less frequent causes in infancy are tetany [108], low blood sugar [106], head injury, and poisoning. From the second half of the first year of age until five or six years of age, convulsions are most commonly caused by infections within and outside of

6 Is a child's age related to the cause of his seizures?

the central nervous system. After six years of age the first convulsion in an otherwise well child is probably idiopathic. Early adolescence is a common time for the first idiopathic seizure to occur.

THE GENERAL COURSE OF DIAGNOSIS AND TREATMENT

7
What diagnostic studies can be done?
Over 600 tests can be done by most medical centers for diagnosis or treatment of conditions related to convulsions. It is obvious, therefore, that some judgment is required to do enough but not too many. Because the child is usually not able to give his own consent to what is done for him, there is a definite responsibility for others to consider carefully what is best for the child.

8
The importance of open communication
The proper evaluation and care of a child with seizures is based not only upon laboratory tests and diagnostic studies, but also upon a fairly thorough knowledge of that child's personality, school performance, medical history, and home environment. Prompt and honest communication between the parents, the physician, the child, and the school will help insure the best possible outcome. Even if the outlook is known to be poor, all of us feel more comfortable and can accept serious conditions if communications have been good.

The evaluation of a chronic disease for which the cause is not clear and the treatment not precise is likely to be difficult to understand. More and more people become involved in complex cases. The combination of uncertainty of outcome, elusive cause, and increasing numbers of interested individuals tends to make communication difficult. Did the psychologist give his opinion to the parents independently, or had he discussed it with the child's physician? Do the child's teachers agree with the parents about their child's intelligence? What opinion does the family doctor have? Does he know about the tests that are scheduled? Who are all these people who seem to know all about the child? What do they do?

The parents and the physician share the responsibility for effective communication. The parents must be honest in giving their information and must share their concern with the physician. The physician will try to keep the parents well informed about tentative diagnoses, scheduled tests, and the introduction of consultants and other personnel. He should be sure that any information given to the parents by others goes along with the general approach already outlined to the parents, except, of course, in those cases where they should be aware of a difference of opinion among these personnel.

Sometimes communications break down completely during a long period of observation and complex studies. Unavoidable problems within the family often upset things. The family may have moved, necessitating a change of family doctors and a new school. There may have been difficult problems within the family which are unrelated to the child's problem but which distract the parents. Perhaps the busy consultant overestimated the parents' grasp of the problem. Whatever the reason, the family is bewildered about what is being done for their child and why. At this point the parents should seek out the one person who seemed to them to have the clearest understanding of the child's problem and the goals of treatment. Together they should redefine the objective, reexamine the working plan, and put things in perspective.

A convulsion is a symptom of an underlying disturbance in the central nervous system. The severity of this symptom, its chances of recurrence, and its influence on later life depend mainly on the basic medical cause. If one knows the medical condition which caused the seizures, an educated guess can be made about the amount of structural or chemical damage produced in the central nervous system. For example, a child who recovers from encephalitis caused by lead poisoning [109] is likely to have suffered some permanent brain damage and will probably need therapy for seizures for many years. Even when the exact cause of the spells is not known, there may be clues which can suggest the scope of the problem in the future. The persistence of definite abnormalities on the electroencephalogram [52], and the continuation of more than one kind of spell in the same individual indicate that the seizures may continue for a long time. Also, certain people seem to have an underlying susceptibility to seizures. An electrical disturbance in the nervous system might cause a seizure in one person who is susceptible, but the identical stimulus might have no effect at all in another person who is less vulnerable. Other factors which influence the general outcome are the age at which the first convulsion occurred, the child's basic intellectual and motor ability, and the possible presence of additional handicaps unrelated to the seizure. Fortunately, seizures generally tend to become isolated and infrequent unless the individual is constitutionally predisposed toward spontaneously recurring attacks. The outlook is not necessarily poor even if seizures begin early in life. The quality of medical care available and community educational facilities will also influence the outcome.

Overall (if children with febrile seizures are included), over 90% of individuals with seizures will never have more than one. Over 50% of children with petit mal will not need daily therapy as adults. Over 30% of children with definite idiopathic seizures will eventually be able to do without therapy. Over 90% of children who are otherwise normal can be maintained spell-free or with no interference with their daily lives with the use of currently available therapy.

10
Convulsions and mental retardation

Although there is no convincing evidence that a convulsion alone causes permanent damage to the brain, it is surprising how many parents and professionals, including some doctors, make this assumption. Some conditions which cause seizures may also produce mental retardation and personality change. In general, however, a change in the personality or competence of a child with a convulsive disorder is related to the child's own feelings about himself and to his reaction to the attitudes of others toward him. A good working rule is to attempt to handle the child as you would any well child of similar age and ability.

11
Adjustment

There is a basic need for adjustment of the child to his parents and his community. Fortunately, the old-fashioned attitudes toward children with convulsions and various neurological handicaps are disappearing. There is a growing positive emphasis on the individual child's potential to contribute to society to the best of his ability. If a child with a chronic convulsive disorder or other long-term neurologic problem senses that the adults around him consider him inferior, he will develop a very poor image of himself. He will not be able to function to the best of his ability *because* he has gotten the idea that people do not expect him to do very well. His parents may either demand too little from him and overprotect him, or they may set unrealistic standards in a defensive effort to prove his ability to others. The successful long-term management of a child with a convulsive disorder is based largely on the development of positive attitudes in him and in all who may come in contact with him.

The consultant's job is to supplement the medical skills which are already available to the child and his family. In most instances the physician selects a consultant who he believes has more experience and training with the type of convulsive disorder that may be present than he himself has. The consultant helps confirm the working diagnosis or alters it if necessary, helps the family select the community resources which are appropriate, and suggests changes in medication as needed. The consultant does not attempt to supplant the physician who is responsible for the child's regular health needs.

**12
The role
of the
consultant**

There are three major goals sought in the successful care of a child with chronic convulsions. His symptoms must be controlled whenever possible; his family must develop realistic expectations, and he must achieve a degree of independence appropriate to his age and ability. The achievement of these objectives often involves a great deal of time and effort on the part of the physicians, the child, his parents, and others, such as his teachers.

**13
General
objectives
of
management**

THE CONSULTATION

Sometimes the first visit to the consultant's office is an unhappy, frustrating experience. The parents are uneasy because their family physician asked for another opinion. Their

**14
The first
visit**

child senses that "something is up" and may be frightened by an unfamiliar office. Each wonders what will happen next. The doctor may use long, complicated words. Many of his questions do not seem to have much to do with the problem. He may suggest some diagnostic tests which sound complicated and expensive. The parents wonder if they are really necessary. The exhausted family may get home and realize they were too tense and upset to understand much of what the doctor said. A great deal of this tension can be avoided if the parents know what to expect in the way of history-taking, physical examination and recommendations. Sometimes the answer can be given after one or two visits. Sometimes a long period of observation and many complex tests are necessary to unravel a problem.

15
The purpose of the medical history
The consulting physician wants to get a complete history of the child's neurological development and general health. He wants a clear picture of that child's environment and personality. He needs to know the family medical background and must get some feeling for the parents' personalities and their expectations for their child. The child's convulsion is a symptom. Perhaps no cause can be found; perhaps a detailed medical and neurological history will provide a clue. The successful treatment of the symptom involves more than medication. The parents, brothers, sisters, and relatives must develop a constructive attitude toward the child's problem. The doctor will be in a much better position to counsel if he knows something about the whole family.

16
The anxious parent
Sometimes a well-meaning individual—often a relative, occasionally a nurse or a doctor—will say of parents, "They are certainly overanxious." Parents should be. They are afraid that something serious may be wrong with their child. They probably have neither the background, the experience, nor the perspective to interpret the symptom which caused them to seek medical help. Parents, however, should recognize their anxiety and try not to let it interfere with what is being done for the child. Perhaps they have read something upsetting in a magazine or newspaper about a child that sounds just like theirs. Sometimes a well-meaning neighbor's thoughtless re-

marks provoke even more worry. Perhaps they do not quite know how to ask the consultant a question. They are afraid; they want to understand but do not wish to appear ignorant. If parents can be honest about their anxiety, and if they can share their concern with the consultant, he can deal with them in a reassuring and constructive way.

The consultant's first questions are aimed at finding out as much as possible about the seizures themselves. He will want to know the date of onset of the first seizure and the exact symptoms. He will want to know if the convulsion has recurred. He will ask about the child's health and surroundings at the time of the first episode; whether he was sick at the time; if there had been any upsetting changes at home or at school.

17 Important details of the medical history

There are some conditions which resemble convulsions but which are not true seizures in that there is no distortion of the electrical discharge from the brain [73–82]. These conditions can be ruled out by skilled and detailed questioning about the exact circumstances and symptoms of the "seizure." Occasionally, an EEG, "a brain-wave test," is·needed to rule them out completely [43–53].

Once the consultant is sure that a true seizure has occurred, he will want a detailed account of the child's medical health starting with the mother's health during pregnancy. The events at delivery are also extremely important. He will also want to know what immunizations the child has received, and he will want to know in general about the health of other members of the family.

After the doctor has obtained a clear picture of the child's symptoms, his general health, his family, and his environment, he must determine whether the seizure occurred in an otherwise normal child. In other words, he must determine the state of that child's mental development in relation to normal expectations for a child of his age. Observant parents can provide many of the important details. Sometimes these observations can be documented. Baby books, family albums, and even home movies are extremely helpful. A child's development may be delayed by prematurity, illnesses, personality,

18 The developmental history

and even environmental opportunity. The big, placid boy will develop more slowly than the busy little girl. Twins are notoriously late talkers. Toddlers who live in some parts of Florida are slow in learning to climb stairs because most homes in that area have no stairs. A deviation from the expected normal development for that age may not mean that anything is seriously wrong, but it does need to be explained.

19
Landmarks of
development
A review of some important landmarks at various ages may be helpful.

Four weeks.   The four-week-old baby is aware of his surroundings. He can lift his head up briefly if placed on his abdomen. He has a clear, but not piercing, cry. He blinks when he hears a sudden noise.

Eight weeks.   A social smile, not to be confused with a smiling movement while the baby is asleep, should be the baby's response to anyone with "warm hands and a warm heart." The smile is the first sign of social awareness, and it is the cornerstone for normal personal-social development in the future. It is an extremely important landmark. About 50% of normal babies smile at four weeks of age; over 90% smile by eight weeks. An explanation is in order for an eight-week-old baby who does not smile in response to friendly stimulation.

Sixteen weeks.   Steady head control should be present in a sixteen-week-old baby. He can reach for and grasp a rattle, and he usually brings it to his mouth. He can laugh out loud and he gets quite excited at the sight of his food.

Twenty-eight weeks.   The seven-month-old baby will have discovered his feet, and he may spend many hours playing with them, putting them in his mouth, or simply waving them in the air. He can roll over front to back and back to front. He can sit up briefly, leaning forward on his hands. He babbles happily.

Forty weeks. At forty weeks the baby has developed the ability to pick up a small object between his thumb and forefinger. He can pull himself up to a standing position by the rail of the playpen or a piece of furniture. He has learned to crawl, hitching himself along on his arms with his legs dragging behind, and he may have learned to creep on his hands and knees. He can wave "bye-bye."

Fifty-two weeks. The yearling can walk with one hand held and can "cruise" along the furniture. He will have two recognizable words in addition to "mama" and "dada." He may have more.

Fifteen months. By now he walks alone and crawls up stairs.

24 months. The two-year-old toddler runs well and walks up and down steps bringing both feet onto the step before proceeding to the next one. He can put together simple sentences.

36 months. The three-year-old runabout goes up stairs placing one foot on each step. He rides a tricycle.

A "neurological examination" sounds like a complicated and difficult procedure. Although the examiner does go through an orderly and systematic check of the child's nervous system, the examination can be informal and even friendly. The doctor will want to check the child's cranial nerves, his way of walking, his reflexes, his coordination, and any unusual movements. He will note how the child plays with a toy, his attention span, whether he uses his right or left eye predominately, whether he is right- or left-handed and right- or left-footed. He notes how well the youngster relates to people and the test situation. At certain ages, two years for example, a definite negative response to much of the examination is quite normal. The doctor may also want to do a rough check on the youngster's mental ability, vocabulary, and reading skill [29–32].

The neurological examination of an infant includes very

20
The neurological examination

careful measurement of the head and chest. The observer will note the proportions of the baby's body and the symmetry of his head. He will check the soft spot on the top of his head. He will see whether his eyes are straight as he looks ahead. He will put the baby in various positions to check on certain righting reflexes present in the very young baby. He will almost certainly try to get the baby to smile back at him.

Any part of an examination which might frighten a child is delayed until after mental ability, motor skill, language, general personality, and behavior have been observed. There are very few procedures which can frighten a child. For example, because a toddler may become upset when the doctor looks down his throat, this part of the examination is usually postponed until the end.

It is often possible to observe a clinical seizure during the course of the examination. A young infant who has minor motor seizures [69] will often demonstrate these attacks when he wakes up or is startled by a sudden noise or bright light. Other children under stress may have a petit mal spell [67]. In some instances, breathing deeply while at rest will produce a typical petit mal spell.

DIAGNOSTIC PROCEDURES

**21
The choice
of
diagnostic
procedures** Now that the history has been taken and the neurological examination done, the consultant has been able to make a working diagnosis. Certain laboratory and psychological studies may be necessary before definite treatment is started. There are hundreds of laboratory tests which may be done to clarify a neurological problem. The consultant has a responsibility to the child, who has no say in the decision, and to the parents, who may have neither knowledge nor perspective, to limit the procedures only to those which are absolutely necessary to reach a medically sound conclusion.

PSYCHOLOGICAL TESTING

22 Recurrent seizures are physical symptoms. Proper medical treatment can usually control the individual spells, but proper total care of a child with seizures must also consider the child as a complete person. It is important to know his intelligence, his approach to learning, his personality, and his feelings about himself. A psychological examination can help him and his family make the best possible adjustment to his condition, whether it is temporary or long-standing.

**22
Why might
my child
need a
psychological
test?**

Unfortunately, many people invariably associate mental retardation with convulsions. Convulsions may or may not be associated with mental retardation. If a child with recurrent spells has normal intelligence, a psychological examination can establish once and for all his intellectual potential. The possible negative attitude of relatives, teachers, and schoolmates can be counteracted.

In some instances the underlying condition that causes the convulsions may be associated with some intellectual slowness. In this case it is equally important to find out exactly what the child can do well and what difficulties can be expected. In this way realistic goals can be set for him both in school and at home.

The doctor often does a few "screening" intelligence tests on the child's first visit [29–32]. These tests are useful but not conclusive unless they are supported by other, more sophisticated tests. The consultant will probably want a more thorough evaluation by a psychologist.

School psychological tests are given primarily to establish a child's educational placement. In other words, in what grade he should be. Total intelligence is much more complicated than the ability to do numbers and read, the primary factors measured by school *achievement* tests. School tests are often given to children in groups, and any one child might not have been at his best on that particular morning. The educational psychologist is interested in what the child can learn. The clinical psychologist is interested in why and how he thinks as well as in what he has learned. School tests are useful as a general estimation of the intelligence of normal children, but an IQ test, individually administered by a trained psychologist is a much more accurate measurement of your child's *intellectual potential*. The records of any school tests are very helpful to the clinical psychologist, and he will usually request the parents' permission to obtain them from the school, but

**23
My child was
tested in
school.
Must it be
repeated?**

he will then evaluate your child individually to determine scientifically *how his mind works.*

24 How will the psychologist test my child? First of all, the psychologist will take as much time as he needs to make friends with the child so that the child can work at his best. The psychologist will have a good idea of the child's medical problem, and he will choose the tests most useful for that particular child, tests that have been proven by experience to be both valid and reliable. In choosing the tests he will take into account the child's age and present developmental level. The psychologist will try to pick the tests most likely to give the answer sought by the physician and the parents. He will talk to the family and will try to get a feeling of their expectations for the child. His analysis of the test results will involve careful consideration of any social, emotional or physical problems present. Most important, the tests will be carried out in the exact way specified by the designers of the test.

25 How should I prepare my child for psychological testing? Children will usually be curious about what kind of doctor they are going to see. You can explain that, while he is called "doctor," he does not given medicine or shots and does not examine you for physical conditions. He is a doctor who talks to and plays with children. A very young child need be told only that "he is going to play some games with paper and pencil and blocks." An older child may be told that he is going to do some tests and puzzles "to see how you feel about things." If the child asks, "What things?" the parent may answer, "school," or "your family," or whatever problem seems most important. A teenager or bright preadolescent may not be satisfied with this explanation. If he is being tested for the first time, he should be told frankly that you, as his parent, know that he has certain problems (school, social, or whatever other difficulties your child is experiencing), and that the psychologist will try to understand these problems and to help him to solve them. If the child has been tested before, he may protest that he has already had all these tests. He should then be told that the psychologist is aware of this and is going to try to see how much progress has been made since the last tests and to identify the areas in which more help is needed.

The test should be given when the child is well and rested. Results obtained from testing an exhausted toddler after a long trip are not likely to be valid. One family I know asked to have their six-year-old son's test scheduled at 9:30 A.M. because he would be most alert and cooperative then. It meant that they would have to start out at 4:00 A.M. The boy slept through the trip even though they did not. A previous test, attempted a 4:00 P.M. after his first visit to the diagnostic center, was worthless because he was worn out and irritable.

Intelligence has been defined as "the capacity to acquire and apply knowledge." (*The American Heritage Dictionary of the English Language*, American Heritage Publishing Company and Houghton Mifflin Co., 1969, p. 862.) According to this definition, intelligence involves many skills. Among them are comprehension, memory, good visual-motor coordination, adequate hearing, perceptive ability, and the capacity for abstract reasoning. Measurement of perception checks the child's ability to recognize forms, spatial relationships, and distance.

> **26**
> **What is intelligence?**

"Why are these three things alike?" One child might answer "Because they are all yellow." This is a correct concrete answer. Another child might answer, "Because they are all fruits." This answer shows an additional capacity to think in abstract terms. Abstract reasoning usually begins to appear at about the age of three years.

The true mental age should reflect all of these skills. Many children develop some of these skills far better and earlier than others. The psychologist does not simply evaluate overall mental ability in the form of a "lump sum" IQ although this is very important. He also makes an accurate profile of the child's abilities in each of the vital skills. Children with perceptual difficulties and difficulties with abstract reasoning may have problems with school work even though their memory, general knowledge, and motivation are satisfactory.

By definition, the IQ, or Intelligence Quotient, is the number **27**

27
What is
an IQ?
found by dividing the mental age, the age at which a certain level of abilities and skills is common, (MA) by the chrono-logical age, the age in years, (CA) and multiplying by 100.

$$\frac{MA}{CA} \times 100 = IQ$$

A ten-year-old child with a mental age of twelve has an IQ of 120, or superior ability. A ten-year-old child with a mental age of eight has an IQ of 80, which is considered slow normal. The normal range of IQ is 90 to 110 and approximately 50% of the population falls within this range.

The term *IQ* equals *intelligence* in the minds of many people. A person with a very high IQ may be very bright, but the significance of an IQ is not nearly that simple. In the first place, exactly how was the MA (mental age) calculated? There are dozens of tests used to determine it. A report of a child's IQ must specify which tests were given. The IQ may change to some extent with age if the child's abilities develop at a faster or a slower pace than the *theoretically* "normal" population of the same age. An IQ may be adversely affected by a poor environment, illness, or by crippling anxiety. At best, it is a shorthand notation of how well that child was thinking on that day.

An IQ is useful because it gives a *general* indication of what might be expected from a child in terms of intellectual achievement. For example a college graduate probably has an IQ of about 120. The mean (average) IQ of high school graduates is 110. Someone with an IQ of 110 has a 50–50 chance of graduating from college. An adult with an IQ of 90 can be expected to perform a job requiring some judgment such as assembling machine parts. A well-adjusted adult with an IQ of 60 can complete significant menial tasks competently on a regular basis. The greater the degree of retardation, the more supervsion is needed.

28
Limitations
of
psychological
testing
No test is perfect. There are many factors which can affect test results even under the best of circumstances.

A child with a physical handicap such as a hearing loss, visual problems, poor coordination, or a speech problem is going to do poorly on some sections of almost any test. The score may be unfairly low because the test standards are set for a normal population without a handicap.

Lack of opportunity may hamper some children. A child who has rarely been allowed to handle a pencil may have trouble drawing circles and squares.

The child's own environment may be quite different from that assumed by the test designer. For example, a Pennsylvania Dutch Amish farm boy who did not learn English until age six is going to be severely limited in vocabulary tests. Perhaps the separation of the child from his parents during the test is so upsetting that he cannot pull himself together to attempt any of the required tasks, or perhaps a child might be receiving some medication which could affect the speed of his responses.

Sometimes these limiting factors are significant. A child who is very fearful or very inhibited in the test situation may have similar trouble adjusting to a classroom situation.

Most experienced examiners can judge the reliability of the test. Rarely, another examiner, perhaps of the opposite sex, will obtain better cooperation and be able to report different results.

A child's convulsive disorder may influence the results of psychological testing unfavorably. For example, as mentioned above, the child's medication may be inappropriate so that he is clumsy or sleepy. He may even have frequent unrecognized seizures which interrupt the examination.

The psychologist's report should be a conscientious summary of the child's knowledge, skills, weaknesses, and personality. It may also contain specific recommendations for education and upbringing [42].

PSYCHOLOGICAL TESTS WHICH MAY BE HELPFUL

Three short "screening" tests often used by the physician to get a rough estimate of the child's ability are the Vineland Social Maturity Scale, the Peabody Picture Vocabulary Test, and the Denver Developmental Screening Test. These tests may be given by individuals who are not psychologists, but

29
Psychological
"screening"
tests

the tests still must be administered in the prescribed way to be valid. Psychologists also may use these tests as part of a more comprehensive examination.

30
The Vineland Social Maturity Scale (VSMS) The Vineland Social Maturity Scale consists of yes-or-no questions, to be answered by a person who knows the child well. The child need not be present. The test reveals the degree of independence reached by the child in the areas of "self-help, self-direction, locomotion, occupation, communication, and social relations." The questions are arranged in order of increasing difficulty according to age. Each yes answer counts as one point. The total score is recorded, and the child's *social age* (SA) is determined from a table. A *social quotient* (SQ) is obtained by dividing the social age by the chronological age and multiplying by 100.

Typical questions for a young child are "Does he pull off his socks?" "Does he unwrap candy?" The parents of a seven-year-old might be asked, "Does he tell time to the quarter hour?" "Does he bathe himself?" "Does he go to bed without help?"

The Vineland Social Maturity Scale has the advantage of simplicity. The questions are developed in a logical way from one age level to the next. Since the questions are carefully balanced for types of skills, any "scatter" will be apparent. A six-year-old might score as expected for his age in areas of communication, but he might be several years behind in locomotion because he has a motor handicap. The time required to give the test is only about fifteen minutes, and, since his presence is not required, it can be given even if the child is sick, tired, or uncooperative.

The Vineland Social Maturity Scale does not measure the *performance* of the child. It gives a quick *impression* of how the child compares with other children his age. The results show at what social age the child is actually functioning. If the child is behind, the results will indicate some area of weakness, but they will not explain why these weaknesses are present. The accuracy of the test depends on the parents' estimate of their own child's ability. Since most parents see their children in the best possible light, there is often an understandable bias present. This bias may also be explored because it gives the examiner an idea of how realistically the parents see their child.

This test provides a quick and simple way to check a child's "vocabulary age." The Peabody Picture Vocabulary Test consists of a series of black-and-white line drawings for which a word is given as a clue. The child is asked to choose, from a group of four pictures, the one which suits the word most accurately. The list of 150 words is arranged in increasing order of difficulty. A three-year-old would be expected to associate "bat" with the proper picture. A ten-year-old would be expected to choose the picture best representing "destruction." The tests ends when the individual misses six out of eight consecutive words. Although the test has no time limit, it can usually be given in fifteen minutes. It requires a friendly atmosphere, a sympathetic examiner and adherence to the standard procedure outlined in the manual. Even children with a short attention span often enjoy the pictures and lose interest only when the words become too difficult.

31
The Peabody Picture Vocabulary Test (PPVT)

Many psychologists prefer more elaborate and detailed tests. They feel that a child who likes books, who has a good vocabulary, and who has been generally verbally stimulated will have an unfair advantage over one who has had no opportunity to develop language skills. The resulting difference in scores does not present a true picture of the basic intelligence of either. A child with poor vision or perceptual difficulties may perform poorly simply because of these problems. On the other hand, a child who has multiple handicaps which interfere with performance on more elaborate tests may do well on the Peabody test.

In general, it is a good test with which to start because the child enjoys it and because it gives a quick indication of ability which may be useful in selecting other tests.

This test is widely used to find out if a child less than six years of age is delayed in any area of development. It is easy to administer and no special training is required to interpret the results. Four "sectors" of behavior are checked. These are gross motor (large muscle movements), fine motor-adaptive (fine muscle movements and skills), language, and personal-

32
The Denver Developmental Screening Test (DDST)

social development. The examiner systematically checks the baby's performance on about twenty activities expected to be present at a given age. Some responses can be obtained by observation; others, by questioning the mother or by direct involvement with the child.

The examiner will observe a nine-month-old baby to see if he walks holding onto furniture. He notes whether he bangs two cubes held in his hands. He listens to his "talking," to see if he actually imitates sounds. He places a toy out of his reach to see if he will work toward it.

A "delay" is a failure by a child on an item if he is older than the age at which 90% of the children pass that item. Normal children will show some scattered successes and failures within the four sectors. A child's performance in a given sector is abnormal if he has two or more delays in that sector.

The test does not give an IQ. Its chief purpose is to alert the examiner to the presence or absence of delayed development. It does not predict intelligence, and other tests must be used to discover the *cause* for any delay observed.

33
Specialized psychological tests
There are many elaborate psychological tests available. Seven of the most commonly used tests are described briefly because questions regarding their selection and administration are frequently asked. Although most of them have excellent manuals which describe how to give and score them, considerable skill and experience are required if their results are to be taken seriously. It is possible, for example, to buy a book on the use of a stethoscope, but the interpretation of the sounds would be open to some question. Do-it-yourself use of a stethoscope or of a specialized psychological test give equally unreliable results. Both need experts.

34
The Wechsler Intelligence Scale for Children (WISC)
This test is used for individual testing of a child rather than for testing a group of children together. It takes about 45 minutes for a seven- to ten-year-old child, and one hour for older children. One part of the test requires primarily verbal skills in the form of questions and answers on general information, comprehension, arithmetic, similarities, vocabulary, and digit span. The second part requires motor performance for picture completion, picture arrangement, block design,

object assembly, and coding. Because the subtests are scored separately, the individual's strengths and weaknesses can be seen clearly by the examiner. Many psychologists feel it is the best single test for seven-to-fifteen-year-old children with IQ levels in the 50–150 range. The scoring is open to relatively little question, and the agreement between different examiners is good.

However, a preschooler may be unfairly handicapped by the method of scoring, and other tests, tailored for children in this age range, are usually used for preschool children.

The Stanford-Binet test is the oldest and best standardized test. Most new tests are compared against it for reliability. The results give a comprehensive picture of performance from two years to adult life. A variety of test questions are asked at each age level. It is most useful in the two-to-eight-year age groups. If the child has a handicap, the whole test usually cannot be given. The validity of the test naturally decreases with the modification needed to give it. Most clinical psychologists supplement the S-B test with other tests of ability and achievement and do not report a single IQ score. This is a result of the Stanford-Binet's reliance on verbal skills as a predictor of school performance. Also, other tests of perceptual ability and personality can be selected which will give more valuable information for the problem at hand.

35 The Stanford-Binet Test (S-B)

This test is used to compare the individual against school grade norms. For example, the child is asked to read single words of increasing difficulty until 12 words in a row are missed. This can usually be done in 5–10 minutes. The arithmetic section takes longer to complete (up to 1 hour at the high school level). It is useful from five years to college and it gives a rapid assessment of learning skill. However, the test does not examine in detail why failures occurred.

36 The Wide Range Achievement Test

"Here are some designs for you to copy; just copy them the way you see them." After these simple instructions have been given, most children over four years of age enjoy reproducing the designs they see. These geometric designs include a diamond and circle, various series of dots, and other shapes

37 Bender Gestalt Test

**37
Bender
Drawings
(Visual-
Motor
Gestalt
Test)**
which are presented in a regular sequence. The designs usually require less than 15 minutes to complete, but there is no time limit. The child sees a design and responds to it. In order to reproduce it properly, he must be able to draw the figure and position it properly on a background. Some children have difficulty in distinguishing one shape from another or may have limited ability in recognizing how the figure they have drawn differs from the original. The experienced examiner can usually identify responses normal for a given age or recognize the possibility of a particular clinical condition which requires further consideration.

**38
The
Draw-a-Man
Test**
This is a popular test for mental age and personality. It can be used for children from about five years of age up to college level. The child is asked to draw a man on a sheet of white paper. This is a fairly simple relaxed, nonthreatening request. The examiner notes how the child approaches the task, what directions he asks for, how he handles the pencil. The test requires only 5 to 10 minutes, yet in this short time the examiner gets some clues regarding the child's personality, how he sees himself (his self-image), his coordination, and his perception of shape.

There are some disadvantages. The drawings may vary tremendously on the basis of the child's past experience. The drawings can be "overread" by an inexperienced examiner, and they may be difficult to interpret if the child has a physical handicap.

**39
The Thematic
Apperception
Test (TAT)**
The Thematic Apperception Test is one of several tests designed to reveal personality rather than mental age. The child is shown a series of drawings and he is asked to make up a story about each picture. These stories reveal what things are important to the child, how he sees relationships between people, and what things cause him anxiety. The test is a useful way to get through a child's defenses or "outer shell." By telling stories about someone else, he unconsciously lets his own thoughts and feelings through. The main disadvantages of the test are that the child must cooperate with the examiner by talking to him and that the test is not formally standardized. It is, therefore, a test relying very heavily upon interpretation.

The test is most useful in children over the age of eight. Similar thematic apperception tests for younger children, such as the "Blacky" test, are also commonly used.

The Rorschach is a personality test. The examiner shows the subject a standardized series of ink blots. The child (or adult) is asked to tell what he sees. When properly given under the best circumstances, the test reveals a comprehensive picture of the subject's personality structure. The ink blots allow the individuality of the subject's response to appear. An experienced examiner will be able to determine strengths and weaknesses in the individual's perception of his world. An inexperienced examiner may focus on the more obvious weaknesses in the subjects's personality, and he may not see the strengths of the personality. The successful administration of this test requires considerable training and experience.

40 The Rorschach (Ink-Blot) Test

The Rorschach takes time. A five-year-old child could take the test in about thirty minutes. A college student could take it in from one to three hours. Further time is needed to score it and interpret the results.

For the past few years there has been increasing interest in the child with "minimal brain-damage," "learning disability" and "cerebral dysfunction." These children may have normal or nearly normal overall intellectual ability, but their weaknesses in certain areas interfere with learning [102–103].

41 The Illinois Test of Psycholinguistic Abilities (ITPA)

The Illinois Test of Psycholinguistic Abilities (ITPA) was developed to identify some of these learning disabilities. The "profile" resulting from the test shows strengths and weaknesses in extremely specialized areas. The rather formidable names given to the subtests indicate the type of information obtained: *auditory reception, visual reception, auditory association, visual association, verbal expression, manual expression, grammatic closure, visual closure, auditory sequential memory, visual sequential memory, auditory closure, and sound blending.* Although these tests sound complicated, an experienced psychologist may find their results very helpful in working out specific learning disabilities in a school-age child. The test is lengthy—it takes over an hour to give. As one might imagine, the psychologist must have special training to administer, score, and interpret it. However, the scores are reproducible by different examiners if the high standards demanded by the test manual are maintained. Since the abilities to read, write, and spell are not tested directly, other ways to measure "graphic learning" or letter forms are usually needed to supplement this test.

42
A psycho-
logical
report

I have described both the simple screening psychological tests and the more complicated specialized examinations. It might be helpful to see how a clinical psychologist might report the results concerning a youngster with convulsions who was having some difficulties in school.

PSYCHOLOGICAL REPORT

Tests Used:

NAME: JOHN JONES   Stanford-Binet Form L-M
DATE OF BIRTH: 10-12-65   Figure Drawings
AGE: 6-4 [6 years, 4 months] Vineland Social Maturity
TESTED: 2-17-72   Scale
                                     Bender-Gestalt
                                     Rorschach
                                     Wide Range Achievement
                                     Test

Reason for Referral:

John was seen for psychological evaluation on referral from Neurology Screening Clinic. He has been under study because of difficulties in adjustment at school and for seizure control. Relevant factors in his background include meningitis at 15 months of age, following which he developed grand mal convulsions. At present, his seizures are well-controlled on phenobarbital. John is currently in first grade in public school, seems to be having difficulty learning, has trouble sitting still, and there are complaints about short attention span.

Behavior:

John was initially seen accompanied by mother and father and after he seemed to become comfortable, he allowed mother and father to leave to wait in the waiting room. John was curious about why he was here and an interpretation was offered as part of trying to understand some of the difficulties in school. He generally seemed a bit tense, moved on his feet rather continuously, and he looked around the room considerably rather than paying attention directly to the examiner. His speech and language seem quite good for his age, he has no problem with articulation or fluency. Gross motor coordination for catching a ball seemed adequate for his age although fine motor coordination in use of a pencil and in dealing with the test materials seemed a little less secure. The relationship quality is good, he is not a behavior problem, and he was generally able to attend and concentrate reasonably well in this one-to-one situation.

Test Results:

John is currently functioning at an average to high-average level of ability with a mental age of six years and eight months, IQ in the 100–110 range. He shows a mild degree of scatter of successes and failures with general excellence in the verbal kinds of tests and somewhat less adequacy in tests where he must copy geometric forms, or things of that nature. He would certainly seem to have adequate intellectual development to proceed through school, however.

His figure drawing is characteristically immature and rather more typical of a child of somewhat younger chronological age, and this likely represents his own insecurity about himself and the mild feelings of inadequacy that appear to be present. Despite his intelligence, John shows some impairment of perceptual motor skills, so that he makes rather more errors in reproducing the Bender Gestalt drawings than would be appropriate for his age. Reflecting this discrepancy is the fact that his reading level on the Wide Range Achievement Test is only at the beginning of the first grade, whereas John is almost two-thirds of the way through his first grade experience. He is able to count successfully and deal with simple mathematical concepts at an appropriate level, however. The Vineland Social Maturity Scale is close to chronological age; he has had some difficulty in learning fine motor skills such as buttoning and tying his shoes, but, other than this, seems to be fairly independent.

John's family seemed to have been able to relate to this situation fairly comfortably without excessive overprotection or excessive demands on him for achievement. They have been able to respond to his needs for support in a positive way. However, the youngster himself is quite able to evaluate the discrepancy between some of his skills and those of his classmates, and his feeling of inadequacy is very realistic.

It would seem that what is needed at this time is some individual help around his perceptual-motor development to aid in these skills so that he can be more successful in his academic work and derive a greater feeling of satisfaction in competition with his peers. He performs adequately enough in gross motor skills that competition at recess, etc., would seem to have been adequate enough in this area. However, John evaluates the quality of his writing and reading to his own detriment.

The recommendations are for individual help around the development of more adequate perceptual-motor skills and continued support by the family in his general emotional development. Prognosis would appear to be quite good for eventual academic achievement.

THE ELECTROENCEPHALOGRAM

43
What is an Electro-encephalogram (EEG)?

In the general discussion on convulsions it was stated that each living cell has an electrical discharge. [1] For reasons which are not yet entirely clear, tiny electrical impulses from groups of nerve cells in different locations of the central nervous system unite and give off a characteristic rhythm. This rhythmical electrical activity can be recorded. The recording is reasonably consistent, so that deviations from the accepted normal pattern can be spotted by a trained person. Just as an electrocardiogram records the electrical impulses given off by the heart, the electroencephalogram, or EEG, records the electrical rhythm of the brain.

44
How is an EEG taken?

Although the term "electroencephalogram" sounds formidable, the procedure is painless and not at all frightening if properly done. It is essential to have a technician who enjoys working with children, and the parents should not hesitate to tell their physician if this is not the case. An EEG is simply a measurement of the electrical discharge given off by the brain cells at specific locations. No electricity whatsoever goes into the child's head. The EEG is purely a measurement. The electrodes which will measure the electrical discharge are attached to wires which are connected to a rather complicated machine which records the "brain waves" on special graph paper. There are two types of electrodes. One is a small needle, the other is a metal plate. The needle is inserted just beneath the skin of the scalp. This type of electrode gives an accurate tracing free from artificial movement, but it is impossible to convince a child that a needle does not hurt. In my opinion, needle electrodes should never be used with children, and their use may be an indication that the laboratory in question prefers not to work with children. My suggestion is to ask your pediatrician to refer you elsewhere.

The child can sit in his mother's lap, or, if he is older, in a comfortable chair, or he can stretch out in his crib. The technician attaches the electrodes to the child's head with a special paste which is easily removed during a shampoo later. The first tracings are taken when the child is awake, relaxed, and comfortable (Figure 1). The technician then tries to get the child to sleep (Figure 2). A sleep recording will minimize the effects of extra movements. A tracing is obtained when he is drowsy and when he is asleep. The technician then may ring a bell or flash a light to bring out certain types of brain waves, being careful not to wake him. At some time during the procedure, when the child is awake and cooperative, the technician may try to get him to breathe in and out rapidly about fifty times to bring out a certain rhythmical discharge. If the first EEG has been a pleasant nonthreatening experience, follow-up EEGs will be no problem.

**45
How should
I prepare
my child
for an EEG?**

The child should receive his regular medication, if any, before the EEG, unless you have been told to omit it. I do not routinely ask that an older child be kept awake all night to be sleepy for the test, but it is helpful to skip an infant's or a toddler's nap. A bottle of formula or milk, a favorite book, a teddy bear, or a "security blanket" will help a great deal in making a little one feel at home during the test. I do not usually give a sedative before the EEG. The extra effort and patience required to have the child fall asleep naturally is rewarded by an EEG free from the distorting effect of the sedative.

**46
What will
the EEG
show?**

The electrodes placed on the scalp to measure the electrical rhythm of the brain are relatively large. Only a small portion of the brain (that closest to the skull) is monitored. The EEG can show the presence of abnormal discharges only from the monitored portion. Some changes on the EEG are unique, so

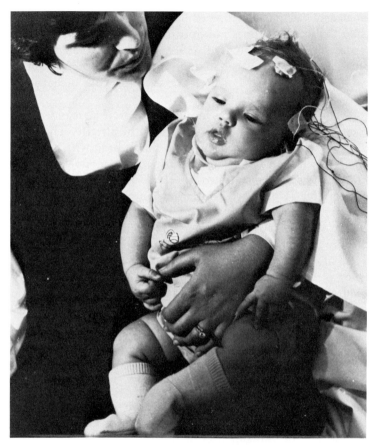

Figure 1. A child being given an EEG. Here the child is awake.

that the electroencephalographer can say "This finding is
usually associated with 'such-and-such' " or that " 'x' percent-
age of patients with a clinical history of thus-and-so have this
finding." However, it is possible for a child with clinical
seizures to have a "normal EEG." In such a case, it is because
the electrodes did not measure the affected portion of the
brain. In other words, an EEG is incapable of measuring a
sufficiently large area of the brain to show the abnormal
activity that probably does occur. It also is not uncommon for
an individual to have an "abnormal EEG" with no clinical
seizures whatsoever.

One could ask what the point is of doing an EEG if it is so inexact. An experienced electroencephalographer studies the number of waves which occur in a unit of time (the *frequency*, [50]) and notes their form. He can raise several diagnostic possibilities. The physician considers his report along with the clinical findings and the results of other diagnostic studies. He often gets confirmation of his working diagnosis from the EEG.

The EEG is often useful in checking on the control of seizures. A child with a history of clinical seizures and an abnormal EEG who has been on medication should have an annual EEG. If there have been no clinical seizures and the EEG is normal, the physician might want to consider reducing the dose or eliminating it altogether. An EEG may also be helpful in identifying a child whose "seizures" may not be real. What may have been accepted as frequent, definite grand

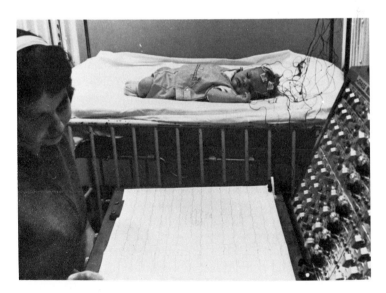

Figure 2. The same child, asleep. This recording is taken so that the effects of extra movements (while the subject is awake) are minimized.

mal seizures [64] may prove to be attempts to attract attention. A normal EEG, particularly during a "seizure" may clarify the situation. On the other hand, sometimes a seriously disturbed child who has made no response to psychiatric care will have EEG findings that suggest serious *organic* disease of the nervous system.

The EEG may show a pattern that suggests a large space-occupying mass such as a collection of blood over the brain. This particular type of EEG is more definite in adults than in children; it is possible for a child to have an accumulation of blood on the brain from an old head injury and have a normal EEG.

The EEG will not always show "brain-injury," "minimal cerebral dysfunction," or "brain-damage." These terms are currently being used loosely, to describe those children of normal or near-normal intelligence who have a learning disability [101–103]. To be sure, *some* "brain-damaged" children have abnormal EEGs with or without clinical seizures, but this finding has very little to do with learning disability. Unfortunately, administrators of some schools are misusing EEGs by making an abnormal EEG a requirement for admission to a class for "brain-injured" children.

47
Interpreta-
tion of the
EEG
The interpretation of an EEG is a highly specialized science. The normal variation among children is considerable, and special training is required to evaluate the tracings. Proper interpretation is most difficult in babies and young children because many rhythms, normal for children, would be definitely abnormal if they were present in an adult.

48
When should
an EEG be
obtained?
The EEG can be abnormal in many conditions, not all of which are at first glance directly related to the nervous system. In some medical centers, EEGs are routinely ordered for children with such conditions as diabetes, congenital heart disease, and thyroid problems. In other institutions, the doctors do not feel that they add a great deal to a solution of the basic problem of these conditions and they are less likely to ask for them. In general, the doctor will ask for an EEG if he feels it will be useful, along with other tests, in the management of the child's condition. An EEG is a legal necessity in most cities

if a head injury involving another party has occurred and loss of consciousness is suspected.

I currently order EEGs for children with the following problems:

1 A repeated loss of consciousness from any suspected cause. The cause might be a seizure disorder, a psychiatric condition, or a heart problem.

2 "Cerebral palsy," with or without a history of seizures [97].

3 Moderate or severe mental retardation.

4 A family history of certain chronic progressive diseases of the nervous system [104].

5 Certain disturbances in body chemistry which can affect the nervous system. Phenylketonuria (PKU) is an example [105].

1929816

6 Suspected brain tumors.

7 Severe learning disability.

8 Psychiatric disturbances such as intractable temper tantrums.

The recording of discharges from the brain is a delicate business. Many conditions affect the results and skilled interpretation is necessary to evaluate them properly. *The EEGs presented in this book are not meant to be used for diagnostic comparisons, but merely to illustrate the wide variations between different types of EEG patterns.*

49
Variations
in the EEG

The EEG has different characteristics at different ages [51]. An "abnormal" finding in one age may be quite normal in another; The state of consciousness will alter the tracing; An artificial sedative will have an effect; Certain drugs, such as the steroids and thyroid extract will change the pattern. It is very important that the individual reading the EEG be aware that the child is taking such drugs. Certain abnormalities in the EEG run in families. What may appear as an electrical distortion can often be found in the EEGs of other members of the child's family and may be of no clinical significance.

The EEG is analyzed for frequency, voltage (amplitude), and form. *Frequency* is the number of waves per second; *voltage* is the measure of the intensity of the electrical discharge (in the case of EEGs, the range is measured in microvolts); *form* is

50
The
EEG
tracing

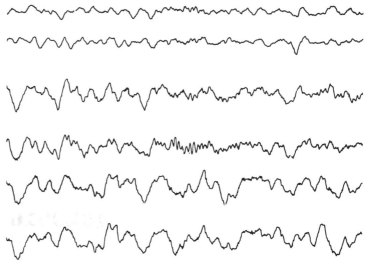

Figure 3. Actual EEG of a normal child.

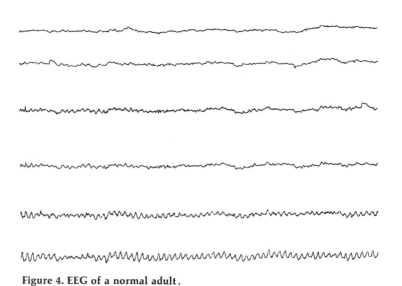

Figure 4. EEG of a normal adult.

the term used to describe the pattern of the discharges as they appear on the written record.

In the newborn period, rhythmical discharges are poorly developed, and the EEG appears rather flat. The EEG of a toddler usually shows random 3-to-7 Hertz waves and some low-voltage fast activity (Figure 3). Gradually, the basic rhythm becomes more regular as the child matures, and by 6 years of age, the pattern is made up mainly of 5-to-7 Hz waves; by 10 years, *alpha* waves (8-to-12 Hz), predominate. During adolescence, some slow wave activity, 6-8 Hz, is not uncommon and may be interpreted incorrectly if adult standards are used. The most common type of rhythm found in the adult, the alpha rhythm, consists of fairly regular waves which occur at frequencies of 6 to 12 Hz, with amplitudes of 20 to 60 microvolts; the second most common is the *beta* rhythm, which has a frequency of 13 to 50 Hz and a lower voltage (Figure 4). Many convulsive disorders are character-

51
The normal EEG at various ages

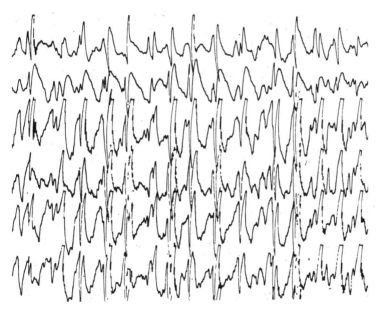

Figure 5. Grossly abnormal EEG. While not all convulsive disorders exhibit this pattern, the neurologist can usually recognize and interpret the distinctive abnormalities that characterize many such disturbances.

ized by markedly abnormal and distinctive EEG patterns, such as that seen in Figure 5.

**52
Abnormal
findings
on the EEG** Most patients with frequent grand mal seizures [60] have definite abnormalities in their EEGs in the intervals between seizures. These consist of random spike discharges, diffuse high-voltage slow waves, or a pattern inconsistent with the child's chronological age. An EEG obtained during a grand mal seizure shows multiple high-voltage spike discharges. An EEG taken right after treatment for the seizure shows a marked change. Patients with infantile myoclonic seizures [65] have a characteristic high-voltage 1–2 Hz spike-and-wave pattern known as *hypsarythmia*. The term is derived from the Greek "hyps," meaning high and lofty. An EEG taken during a petit mal attack shows another kind of characteristic spike-and-wave pattern.

**53
A
perspective
on EEGs** An EEG must be taken carefully and read meticulously with attention to many variables. An EEG alone is not sufficient to establish a diagnosis of a convulsive disorder. However, in most cases an abnormal EEG along with appropriate clinical findings indicates such a condition. It can be an extremely important diagnostic tool when properly used and evaluated.

SOME OF THE OTHER STUDIES

**54
The choice
of studies** Most children with convulsions who are referred for further study receive an EEG, and many undergo some sort of psychological testing. There are, in addition, certain other diagnostic tests which may be helpful. Some of these have a direct bearing on the problem of why the child has spells, others are a check on general health. As always, the choice of tests and their number should be guided by the needs of the individual child rather than by any preestablished routine.

**55
The complete
blood count
(CBC)** A complete blood count can be obtained from a drop or two of blood taken from the finger. In an infant, the heel is often used. The blood count might reveal an unsuspected anemia. Some drugs used in the treatment of convulsions [90, 91] may cause changes in the number of blood cells present. It is there-

fore wise to know the child's blood count before treatment is started. A drop of blood may also be examined for sickle cells. While sickle cell anemia is not a *common* cause of convulsions, it remains a diagnostic possibility in a black child who has had a convulsion followed by weakness in an arm or leg.

Analysis of a urine specimen is another means of checking the general health of the child. The physician tracking down the cause of the child's convulsions will also be looking for evidence of kidney disease [107]. Special tests specifically related to convulsions can also be done on random specimens in the office. The doctor might check for the presence of phenypyruvic acid, found in PKU [105]; excessive coproporphyrin, found in lead poisoning [109]; and acetone, found in ketotic hypoglycemia [106]. More sophisticated tests are done on specimens collected over a period of 24 hours. This type of test might be done to check on amino acids, which could be elevated in lead poisoning and various kidney diseases. Such analyses are best done by a specially equipped laboratory.

**56
Routine
urinalysis**

Convulsions may be caused by many types of distortions in body chemistry. Some are relatively common, some are rare. Usually only a small sample of blood is required.

**57
Blood
chemical
determina-
tions**

A "fasting blood sugar determination" is quite often done to see if a child's spells could be caused by low blood sugar [106]. During periods of stress or fasting, the amount of sugar (also known as glucose) in the blood may drop to subnormal levels. In some susceptible children, low blood sugar may cause a seizure. Unfortunately, the result may not have much validity unless the specimen is taken during a seizure— the body's regulatory system may respond so quickly that the blood sugar value may be normal soon after the spell. A single normal fasting blood sugar test does not exclude the diagnosis of low blood sugar. More complicated tests involving several blood sugar determinations over a period of time may be needed.

A "blood (or serum) urea nitrogen determination" is a general analysis of the state of the kidneys. It is a little more sensitive than a routine urinalysis.

Defects in the body's use of calcium may also be associated with seizures [108]. If a low calcium level in the blood is

suspected clinically and if the level obtained by testing borderline, special tests are sometimes used to check on the body's
response to the calcium regulating hormone.

Other less common chemical diagnostic tests are determination of: lead level to check on lead poisoning [109];
phenobarbital and Dilantin levels to check on therapy and
possible overdose of these drugs; and amino acid levels for
such specific conditions as PKU [105].

58
The x-ray
studies

The physician will almost always order an x-ray examination
of the skull if a diagnosis of a recurrent convulsive disorder
is seriously being considered. In most instances no abnormality
will be found, a fact which may not be appreciated by parents
who expect to be told the results quickly. Rarely, deposits of
calcium from a previous injury or infection, evidence of a
brain tumor, or some other unexpected condition may be
found.

X-rays to determine bone age may be helpful. The bones
of the body develop in an orderly, standard sequence throughout childhood and adolescence. This development can be affected by chronic disease. Examination of the bones may
show evidence of lead poisoning, rickets, or other disturbances
in the body's use of calcium.

59
Air-studies
(Pneumoen-
cephalogram)

The purpose of an air-study (pneumoencephalogram or air
encephalogram) is to demonstrate the location of a neurosurgically correctible condition. This is done by removal of
spinal fluid and by replacing it with an equal amount of air.
Because the density of air differs from that of tissue, the skull
x-ray taken after the air is injected will reveal the various cavities of the brain known as ventricles. If a tumor, old blood clot,
or cyst is present, its size and accessibility can be determined
from the x-ray films. All children who have an idiopathic
convulsive disorder, idiopathic mental retardation, uncomplicated reading disability, and most forms of cerebral palsy have
normal air studies or common abnormalities for which there
is no neurosurgical treatment. Practically all of these conditions can be identified by other means so that a potentially
hazardous procedure can be avoided. Unfortunately, the decision concerning the wisdom of doing the air study presents

itself to the parents at a difficult time. After the procedure is done and nothing is found, many parents are critical both of the cost of the procedure and the child's headache and psychic discomfort. In childhood, the probability of a brain tumor causing only seizures—without other signs, symptoms, or history which are apparent from office procedures—must be very small.

The risk of death from anesthesia is relatively low in children (only one in one thousand), but it does exist. Headache, nausea, and vomiting may persist for two or three days after the procedure. The incidence of infection and other serious after-effects is low. How frequently emotional difficulties begin with or are made worse by any procedure is not known.

60
Angiography

This procedure should be done if a neurosurgically correctible defect is thought to be present. A decision concerning whether an angiogram, an air-study, or both should be done in a particular clinical situation is a matter of surgical judgment. Factors which must be included are the following: The skill and experience of the surgeon, the facilities at his disposal (including x-ray equipment, anesthesia), and the child's condition. The procedure consists of injecting a special dye into a blood vessel. The passage of the dye into the blood vessels of the brain is recorded by x-ray film at regular intervals. If the blood vessels are filled in an abnormal fashion, the reason may be a correctible neurosurgical defect. Complications for young children may be complications of anesthesia, injury to the blood vessel in which the dye is placed (with possible transient and, rarely, permanent damage), or, rarely, a reaction to material used in the dye.

61
Brain scan

A scan is also used when a neurosurgically correctible defect is thought to be present. The test is done by the administration of a small amount of radioactive material into a vein. The distribution of material as it circulates within the brain is counted and a density graph is made. An unusual amount of uptake indicates a mass which might be amenable to surgery. This is a very safe procedure (by today's standards) and can be helpful.

**62
Echoen-
cephalogram**

This test is done when the doctor suspects that a blood clot or brain tumor in one half (hemisphere) of the brain has crowded the other hemisphere into a smaller space. In some instances, ventricular size can be determined. The device is a small sonar. It is relatively easy to operate and it is painless. A sound impulse is sent across the brain and its echo recorded. When it strikes a tissue of different density, change in the echo occurs. By comparing the two halves of the brain with each other and with previous experience, some conclusions can be drawn.

PART TWO

Convulsions and Their Treatment

"FITS" AND FAINTS

The parents of a child who has convulsions are understandably eager to obtain definite answers to certain questions: How often, if ever, will the spells recur? How long will the child need to take medication? Will the spells have any permanent effect on the child's intellect or personality? Unfortunately, the answers to these questions are by no means clear-cut. Various types of abnormal electrical discharges from the brain will produce characteristically different convulsive symptoms. There are many known causes for convulsions, and many that remain unknown. The outlook and duration of treatment may depend on the type of seizure the child has and on the underlying cause, if known. Often the management of the convulsions is minor in relation to the overall treatment of the basic cause. There are numerous other factors to consider. The age of the child, his reaction to medication, and even his family environment can affect the outcome. The following discussion of each type of convulsion must be offered therefore as nothing more than a general approach. There are no final answers.

**63
An approach
to the
problem**

TYPES OF SEIZURES

A grand mal convulsion is the most common type of seizure. It is also the most frightening to a parent or onlooker. Some children may have a period of irritability or headache before

**64
Grand mal
seizures**

the onset of a convulsion, but this preliminary warning or "aura" is much less common in children than in adults. The child usually stiffens suddenly and falls to the ground; he becomes quite pale; his eyes roll upwards and their pupils dilate; his head is thrown backward; he may give a peculiar shrill cry as air is forced out by a sudden contraction of the diaphragm. Sometimes there is a loss of bladder control. The child's face becomes red, then it turns gray as breathing ceases for 20 to 40 seconds. This generalized stiffening, or *tonic*, phase is followed by the *clonic* phase of rhythmic contraction of the arms and legs. In this stage, the child's color improves, he begins to breathe, and generalized jerking movements occur. After a few minutes these movements cease and the child awakens. He may be a little confused, and he will frequently have a headache. He usually will want to sleep for several hours afterwards. Occasionally, a convulsion may occur at night while the child is asleep. An older child may awaken with a headache, and he may not have any clear recollection that anything unusual happened.

First aid for a grand mal seizure consists mainly of preventing injury to the child. Tight clothing around the neck should be loosened. He should be rolled on his side and a soft object such as a coat should be put under his head. He should be moved away from any objects which might injure him. *It is useless to try to put anything between the teeth.* If the tongue is bitten, it will have happened during the early tonic stage of the spell. Forcing the mouth open risks injury to the teeth and provides extra unnecessary stimulation. The atmosphere surrounding the child should be one of reassurance and calm.

Occasionally, grand mal seizures occur repeatedly every few minutes. The name "status epilepticus" is applied to this situation. It is usually caused by a failure to take medication as prescribed. *Status epilepticus is a medical emergency.* After first aid has been given, the child should be taken to a hospital for medical treatment.

Grand mal seizures occur at any age from early infancy up through adult life. Most grand mal seizures are *idiopathic*— no cause can be found for them. Idiopathic grand mal seizures commonly begin to occur during adolescence. There are, how-

ever, also many definite organic causes [4, 5]. A febrile convulsion [65] is a grand mal convulsion associated with fever,
and is not uncommon in early childhood.

Grand mal seizures can be treated with many different
drugs. Phenobarbital alone, or in combination with Dilantin,
is the most satisfactory medication, in my experience [86, 88].

Most children with seizures should receive anticonvulsant
medication for a considerable period of time. It is best to avoid
predicting how long any particular child will need to take the
medicine since the physician has no way of prejudging the
child's response to medication or the severity of his condition.
It is much better to maintain small doses of medication for a
long period of time than to stop the medication and have a
recurrence of seizures. Recurrence of seizures signifies failure
in the minds of the parents, creating an atmosphere of pessi-
mism and frustration that can complicate the child's treatment.
The EEG is useful for judging the need for therapy. A child
whose EEG remains abnormal while on adequate medication
is obviously going to need that medication. The longer the
period during which the child continues to have occasional
spells, the longer the period of treatment. Very few children
who have several grand mal spells in childhood "outgrow"
them without medication.

Medication is prescribed in terms of body weight [87]. As
the child grows, he weighs more. In some children, it is necessary to increase medication as the child grows, not because
his condition is worse, but because the dose should remain
constant in terms of body weight. Other children might be
maintained on the original dose even though they continue
to grow and gain weight. These children are actually taking
a smaller dose because the amount of drug stays the same but
the number of pounds increases.

The outlook for control of grand mal seizures is good,
provided there are no associated handicapping conditions. The
child who receives prompt, adequate treatment after only one
or two seizures, whose seizures do not recur, whose EEG
remains normal, and whose medication remains at the same
dose has an excellent outlook.

The first year of management of a child with grand mal
seizures is one of careful observation. If the working diagnosis

is "idiopathic convulsions" it might take at least a year to be sure the spells are indeed idiopathic and that they are unrelated to any organic condition. The child's response to dosage of medication must be carefully evaluated. After this initial period of observation, management passes into the maintenance stage. Now that the spells are under control, the doctor can check on the youngster's total environment, including his home and school. The best possible therapeutic result will be obtained when the diagnosis is made accurately, the proper medication is properly given, and the child's total environment is as right for him as circumstances will allow.

65
Febrile
seizures

A febrile seizure is a grand mal convulsion associated with fever produced by an infection outside the central nervous system. Throat infections, ear infections, and roseola or "baby measles" are common febrile conditions producing this type of seizure. Sometimes the convulsion occurs at the height of the fever; sometimes it occurs just before the temperature rises. A simple febrile convulsion rarely occurs for the first time in a child over the age of three years. The physician will undoubtedly make sure that the fever is indeed caused by an infection outside the central nervous system rather than by a more serious condition such as encephalitis or meningitis. A simple febrile convulsion is usually short and of no great significance, although it is a very alarming episode for a parent to witness.

It is difficult to estimate the incidence of febrile convulsions because so many are never reported, but a reasonable estimate might be that one out of 30 children has a history of one or more febrile convulsions. Parents, of course, want to know if there is a chance of the child's developing chronic nonfebrile convulsions later on. The answer to this question is not entirely clear. There is little evidence that a febrile convulsion will, in itself, predispose a child to chronic convulsions later. But a significant number of persons with chronic recurrent convulsions have a history of febrile seizures in early childhood—one must keep in mind, however, that only those with chronic seizures were *asked* if they had ever had febrile seizures.

Sometimes a child will have more than one febrile convulsion. The physician and the family may become concerned that the problem may be more complicated than was previously thought. Because simple febrile convulsions normally are harmless and of no great significance, they need no detailed investigation. When, then, should definitive studies be undertaken? The "rule of three" may be helpful as a general guide. Any child who has more than three febrile convulsions or who has one febrile convulsion over the age of three years deserves a thorough investigation for other basic causes.

An EEG taken shortly after a febrile convulsion may remain abnormal for up to a week or it may be completely normal. It does not provide any particularly useful information after a single simple febrile spell, but it may be helpful in assessing whether or not a chronic disorder is present, if taken at least two weeks after the most recent of several febrile convulsions.

Treatment of the febrile convulsion consists of reducing the temperature as quickly as possible by such measures as sponging with cool water and administration of appropriate doses of aspirin. Some physicians routinely prescribe an anticonvulsant dose of phenobarbital to be given at the very onset of the fever. Most suggest prompt administration of aspirin at the beginning of any illness, such as a cold, which may later be complicated by fever. If the fever can be prevented, the convulsion will not occur. A few physicians feel that it is necessary to give a child with a history of one or more simple febrile seizures a daily maintenance anticonvulsant dose of phenobarbital. There is a considerable difference of opinion about this therapy.

A convulsion in a newborn infant (under 30 days old) is quite hard to detect. The obvious tonic (stiffening) and clonic (visible rhythmical) movements that characterize grand mal seizures [64] are rarely apparent during a baby's first few weeks. A newborn baby may have a convulsion consisting of a short episode of stiffening followed by a few jerking movements of an extremity. If one watches the infant closely, one may see the baby's eyes move rapidly, his skin become pale, his muscles become unusually weak, and note the presence of awkward jerking movements. Sometimes the infant's breath-

**66
Seizure
in the
newborn
period**

ing becomes slow and irregular, and the neck and back become rigid. There may be a weak cry; the pupils enlarge, and chewing movements occur.

The electrical activity of the brain in a newborn infant is poorly developed, but abnormal changes may be recorded. Even though an EEG is technically difficult to obtain in a newborn baby, it may be the only objective means of detecting a seizure. Sometimes simultaneous EEG recordings and motion pictures are helpful.

The presence of a seizure in the newborn period suggests some sort of damage to the brain. Lack of oxygen and glucose before, during, and after delivery must be considered, as must infection of the central nervous system. An infant who has such an infection will usually also be drowsy, unstable, or have other symptoms. Other causes of seizures in the newborn are low blood sugar, low blood calcium, and insufficient amounts of vitamin B6 (pyridoxine). An infant born to a mother who is addicted to heroin will also be addicted and will have withdrawal symptoms which resemble seizures. Whatever the cause, good general care including prevention of shock, appropriate sedation, and maintenance of breathing are essential.

The outlook for future normal development in a newborn baby who has had convulsions depends of course on the basic cause and the extent of any damage to the brain.

If the family history is free of nervous system disease, if the mother's general health has been good, if the obstetrical history is normal, if the infant is of normal weight and appears normal in every other way, and if the seizures occur before the third day of life and are of brief duration, the outlook is usually best. Many babies who are seriously ill during the newborn period receive optimal care and go on to become perfectly normal adults. Long-range predictions are not really very accurate for this age group. In general, the better the care, the better the outcome.

67
**Petit mal
seizures**
The symptoms of petit mal convulsions can be very slight and pass almost unnoticed. During the most common form of petit mal the child stops what he is doing. His eyes roll upward, his lids flicker and his head nods rhythmically for less

than 15 seconds. He may then smile briefly. During this time he has a momentary lapse of consciousness. For example, a child may stop while taking a drink of water, have a brief spell, and continue to drink as if nothing had occurred. Occasionally there is an associated jerking movement of the body or arms. Petit mal rarely occurs below three years of age, and is more common in girls. In most instances the cause of petit mal is unknown.

The EEG of a child with petit mal is quite characteristic. It shows spike and wave forms occurring with a frequency of 3 Hz [52]. Sometimes this particular abnormality and the accompanying spells may be brought about by having the child breathe deeply and rapidly. Relatives may also have similar EEG findings, even if no seizures have occurred.

Treatment for simple petit mal is relatively effective. Zarontin, alone or with phenobarbital, is widely used [86, 91]. A child who has very little involuntary movement below the neck during a spell is often the easiest to control. A neurologically normal ten-year-old girl of normal intelligence who has had the seizures for only a short time, who has a characteristic EEG and who responds promptly to medication has a good chance of becoming seizure-free. The outcome may be less favorable if the petit mal spells are associated with movements of the arms, legs, or trunk, if significant mental retardation is present, or if the seizures followed brain infection or injury. About half the children with petit mal go on to develop grand mal or psychomotor seizures later.

A psychomotor seizure may be defined as a complicated but **68** inappropriate involuntary motor act which occurs in a state of **Psychomotor** altered consciousness. The symptoms are extremely variable **seizures** and they may be hard to recognize. Perhaps a young child will have a slight *aura*, or warning. He may cry out or run for help. He is usually pale, especially around the mouth. He may hold out one arm, make a slow half-turn to the side, and fall to the ground. Occasionally a child will remember that he was sitting at a table, but afterward, he finds himself standing by a door and has no recollection of how he got there or of how long he has been standing there. A child might become vague and confused while playing and might destroy a favorite toy. After a nap of an hour or two he awakens, completely normal, and is outraged over the destruction of his plaything.

Psychomotor seizures may occur at any age after two years. Specific causes have not been established and most cases must be considered idiopathic in origin. The EEG may be normal before and shortly after a spell, so that diagnosis is even more difficult. If an EEG could be obtained during a spell, it would show various nonspecific abnormalities. Although drug control is less effective than in grand mal and petit mal, phenobarbital and diphenylhydantoin are usually satisfactory. The drugs Mysoline and Mebaral [89, 92] can also be used to control psychomotor seizures.

A satisfactory therapeutic result is dependent on the severity of the convulsive disorder. A child who has no subsequent seizures after the prompt initiation of therapy will do well. Some children with psychomotor seizures require fairly large amounts of medications and some have other types of seizures as well. Satisfactory control for psychomotor seizures mixed with another type may be difficult.

**69
Minor motor
seizures
(infantile
myoclonic
seizures)**

Minor seizures (that is, seizures of short duration) may be difficult to recognize and describe. If a series of seizures occurs it may be possible to call another adult to witness them. In a few minutes, however, the baby may appear quite normal. A parent may be concerned because the infant seemed to be in pain and drew his legs up on his abdomen. During this episode, he may have appeared unusually wide-eyed, alert, and easily startled. In another form of minor motor seizure, the mother might notice that her baby suddenly drops his head forward and jerks his arms upward. Sometimes, parents may be certain that something is amiss, but they may have difficulty convincing their family and physician. Delay in recognition of minor seizures is unfortunate because successful treatment in a previously normal child may depend upon prompt diagnosis and administration of medication.

Minor motor seizures occur between the ages of three months and two years. They are commonly associated with a basic congenital abnormality of the brain or with a chronic progressive disease of the nervous system. Some previously normal children demonstrate minor motor seizures after an episode of encephalitis which might have been quite mild.

The EEG may show a very characteristic pattern known as hypsarhythmia [52]. The presence of this abnormality has a serious implication for subsequent development.

In my experience, the most satisfactory treatment is the administration of adrenocorticotropic hormone, although there is a considerable difference of opinion about the proper therapy for minor motor seizures of young infants.

The results of treatment in minor seizures are variable. A baby with a congenitally damaged brain or with an insidiously progressive disease is not going to do well whatever the treatment. A previously normal child who has an onset of seizures near two years of age and who receives very prompt diagnosis and therapy may develop normally. However, many of these children may have learning disabilities or cerebral dysfunction later on [101–103]. These learning difficulties may be related to the encephalitis which produced the spells rather than to the spells themselves.

70 Akinetic seizures

An akinetic ("without motion") seizure starts suddenly. The child may fall and stiffen his arms. Then he drops forward onto his hands and knees, but he does not shake. The spell usually lasts between 10 and 60 seconds. A child might or might not go to sleep afterward. An EEG of a child with this type of seizure usually shows slow spikes and waves of less than 3 Hz. In most instances the akinetic type of seizure is associated with a basically abnormal brain (a condition that existed at birth) or a chronic disease of the nervous system. The spells are often successfully controlled by Mysoline and phenobarbital [86, 92], but treatment of the underlying cause remains a problem.

71 Reflex seizures (environmental)

Reflex seizures are produced by various types of stimulation such as light, touch, pain, smell, or simply reading or hearing music. The only stimulating sensation which has not been reported is taste. The seizures are quite dramatic, but they often respond well to anticonvulsant medication.

Techniques which gradually condition the individual to accept a milder but similar stimulus without having a seizure are being used successfully. With this method it is possible to increase the number and intensity of the stimuli gradually, until the kind of stimulus which previously caused a seizure can be tolerated. The conditioning, after it has been once obtained in the hospital, can be maintained at home in a variety of ways. For example, a child for whom flickering light induces a seizure can be conditioned by repeated exposure to a flashing light that appears to grow brighter. After the child is taught to tolerate the flashing light, a clicking sound is introduced as a secondary conditioning stimulus. The child can maintain the conditioned state at home by wearing especially designed glasses. These are constructed so that a click sounds behind the ear whenever light fails to fall on the photocell built into the front of the glasses. By passing the outspread fingers between a light source and the photocell, the clicks can be made to occur. Routine exercises several times daily can maintain the "conditioning." Other, similar techniques for preventing reflex seizures due to voice, music, and other stimuli have been successful in meeting the needs of the individual.

One child with reflex seizures suddenly developed rhythmic and symmetrical movements of his arms accompanied by brief lapses of consciousness, whenever he was touched on the head. Seizures did not occur unless he was touched on the head. His EEG showed a spike-and-wave pattern. His seizures stopped entirely after anticonvulsant therapy consisting of phenobarbital was started. This type of seizure is relatively rare.

72
Self-induced
seizures
It is possible for some children with convulsive tendencies to learn how to induce a seizure. This kind of behavior is often difficult to manage by drugs alone; psychiatric help may be required. In some instances the child may seem to enjoy the escape or the sensation associated with the seizure and use it as a mechanism for relief of tension and anxiety. The most common self-induced seizure is petit mal produced by flickering light, but other types of seizures may be brought on by children with convulsive tendencies of various types. In some clinical situations the difference between an idiopathic seizure and a seizure brought on by a certain set of circumstances is not clear. On occasion the occurrence of the seizure seems to be associated with conscious or subconscious attempts to manipulate the parents. Take, for example, the case where a

mother plans to leave her child with a relative for a few days; she mentions that the child will probably have a seizure during this period. The youngster, who is susceptible to self-induced seizures, quite predictably has one. After this type of episode has been repeated several times, the mere preparations for leaving the child can bring on a true convulsion. This kind of incident may represent a coincidence, but until more information is available, the extent of environmental influence remains a highly controversial issue.

A light-induced seizure may be brought on by having the child look at a bright light and move his hands in front of his eyes, or blink, until a spell occurs. A child may look at oncoming headlights while riding in a car at night and use the post of the windshield or trees to interrupt the light thereby bringing on a seizure. One child who had a petit mal seizure whenever his parents' car reached a particular point in the road, seemed to look forward to that part of the journey.

Some children with self-induced light seizures have been known to set a television screen so that it flickers. There are even some children who will be sensitive to a flickering black and white television picture but not to one in color.

CONDITIONS RESEMBLING SEIZURES

A few conditions which occur in childhood are characterized by drowsiness, confusion, and even unconsciousness. These disorders are often recurrent and each recurrence is accompanied by a specific set of symptoms for each individual child. Sometimes there are also mild distortions of the electroencephalographic pattern. Some physicians feel these conditions may represent a form of a convulsive disorder.

There really is no point in worrying about whether a condition such as childhood migraine is a form of a convulsion or not. The problem is quite individual for each child, and successful management often depends more on the patient's temperament, environment, and health rather than on the specific EEG abnormality. In general, treatment should be directed toward *the child*, not the EEG.

CONDITIONS OF UNCERTAIN NATURE

73
Migraine Tommy, just six, returned from his first day in first grade complaining of a mild headache. His mother noticed he was quite pale, and she suggested that he take a rest. He dozed off almost immediately, but he awoke fifteen minutes later with a severe headache over his entire forehead and he said his stomach hurt. He went back to sleep again, but he awoke in a few minutes with the same headache and greater pain in his stomach. He vomited. His color returned, and he fell into a deep sleep. He awoke two hours later feeling completely well. He had a vague recollection of being sick, but he remembered very few details. He had never had any symptoms like this before.

Both his parents had occasional tension headaches, and his father also had had a history of migraine headaches through adolescence.

Tommy continued to have attacks about every six weeks during that school year, often on a Friday. His mother quickly learned the symptoms of an impending attack. She consulted her family physician. He gave Tommy a thorough examination. The doctor advised her to be friendly and sympathetic but not to hover over the child. During attacks, she reassured Tommy that he would feel better in a short time, and she did her best to make him comfortable in a casual way. Tommy, the youngest of three boys, was conscientious and always tried to do his best. His mother also worked closely with his teacher to minimize the stresses of first grade. At home she and her husband made a conscious effort to let Tommy know that they loved him and accepted him as he was and that he need not try so hard to please them or keep up with his brothers.

During the year, the attacks diminished in severity. He had no attacks during the summer. During the following winter he had only two attacks, although he did have an occasional very mild headache when he was tense or tired.

This little boy had one form of childhood migraine. The symptoms are not as clear-cut as they are in adults, and nausea, vomiting, and abdominal pain are more pronounced. An EEG taken during an attack is usually abnormal. Some children can be helped simply by minimizing stress and fatigue; others need daily anticonvulsant doses of pheno-barbital as well. The mechanism underlying migraine is not well known, but it is known that it is the sudden narrowing of the blood vessels triggered by stress or fatigue that causes the pain. The resultant diminished blood supply may cause distortion of the electrical discharge of the brain cells and may account for the drowsiness and occasional confusion.

Some children have recurrent episodes of severe abdominal pain followed by periods of sleep. The unfortunate term "abdominal epilepsy" has been used to describe these symptoms. Recurrent abdominal pain followed by sleep is almost always accompanied by headache and nausea. This type of episode is a form of childhood migraine, and not a true form of epilepsy.

74 "Abdominal epilepsy"

A child with the symptoms of narcolepsy has a sudden, overpowering desire to sleep during the day. The desire often comes on at odd times, such as while the youngster is involved in some activity such as walking or talking. The child ceases what he is doing and "falls in a heap" into a light sleep from which he can be easily aroused. He is alert rather than confused afterwards. The condition may be brought on by emotional upsets, or it may be associated with a variety of central nervous system conditions, or no cause at all may be found. The condition is very rare in childhood but it must be properly diagnosed and differentiated from genuine seizures of the akinetic type. [70].

75 Narcolepsy

NONCONVULSIVE CONDITIONS

Children and adults who lose consciousness for any reason often look pale and have a few random jerking movements.

Unlike migraine and narcolepsy, which might be considered forms of convulsion by some physicians, these conditions are not convulsions at all. They are included because they must be carefully differentiated from a true seizure.

76 Simple fainting A person "blacks out" and falls over when the blood supply to the brain is suddenly diminished. Sometimes the normal blood supply to the brain collects in the organs of the body during prolonged standing, and circulation to the head is sluggish. Soldiers of the Buckingham Palace Guard are said to contract their calf muscles periodically while standing, in order to keep the blood flowing. Sometimes there is a reflex pooling of the blood in the body in response to an emotional shock or an uncontrolled primitive fear such as the sight of blood or the insertion of a needle into a vein for medical reasons. Boys, girls, men, and women are all vulnerable to fainting spells. Each person has his own threshold for "blacking out." This threshold is partially determined by temperament and general health. Proper treatment, of course, is to place the individual in a horizontal position or with feet slightly elevated until the blood supply to the head is restored to normal. Individuals with certain types of heart disease are also subject to fainting attacks. These individuals faint because the heart temporarily cannot pump enough blood to the head. This type of attack, of course, also requires treatment of the basic heart condition.

77 Loss of consciousness during swimming A far more serious type of loss of consciousness can occur during competitive swimming as a result of sudden oxygen depletion. For some reason, competitors in the breast stroke are especially vulnerable. Some swimmers, often experts, breathe deeply, exhaling carbon dioxide, before plunging underwater. The carbon dioxide content of the blood (which ordinarily stimulates the respiratory center of the brain) is thereby diminished, and a swimmer may lose consciousness when the body's oxygen runs low. There is, of course, a vast individual difference in the amount of oxygen depletion necessary to produce loss of consciousness.

This type of near-drowning may superficially resemble a convulsion. Before the swimmer's breathing is restored by

artificial respiration, he may jerk his arms and legs rhythmically. Onlookers could mistakenly assume by this that the
swimmer had a convulsion and then lost consciousness. This,
of course, is not the case. People who have chronic convulsions
and whose seizures are under reasonable control very rarely
have any difficulty while swimming [116].

A child who has emotional problems and who may have had
one or more genuine convulsions can have hysterical episodes
which superficially resemble grand mal seizures. He may have
overheard descriptions of his spells or of someone else's. For
reasons that are not always clear, he can work himself up
into giving a good imitation of an actual seizure. A child in a
hysterical attack has a flushed face which never turns pale; his
eyes often remain closed. If his eyes open, his pupils do not
dilate. Jerking movements are consciously produced in such a
way as to avoid injury. Bladder control is not usually lost and
rambling disconnected moans and fragments of conversation
are common. Treatment, of course, is directed toward the
underlying psychologic disorder.

**78
Hysteria**

One of the most common forms of loss of consciousness in
childhood is breath-holding.
     Larry, an exuberant three-year-old, ran up a steep hill to
tell his mother some exciting news. As he reached the top,
he stumbled onto his knees, opened his mouth to cry and
suddenly lost consciousness for about ten seconds. He woke
up, cried for a minute, then told his mother his news. A
similar episode happened a month later after a bout of loud
crying brought on by a fall downstairs. Careful examination
by his family physician found nothing unusual at all. His
mother was told that he had a tendency to black out after
slight oxygen loss such as that following sudden severe
exercise or intense crying. He told her this was not unusual
in early childhood and that Larry would grow out of it. He
did.
     Patrick, a determined four-year-old lost consciousness
for the first time after a severe temper tantrum at the age of
two. His immature 21-year-old mother was terrified and a
great deal of fuss was made over the episode in the family.

**79
Breath-
holding**

Patrick, who was as perceptive as he was stubborn, soon realized that he could throw his mother into a tailspin by putting on a temper tantrum and holding his breath until he passed out. He then found that he could get what he wanted by simply *threatening* to hold his breath. He rather enjoyed making demands in the supermarket for special goodies, shrieking "I'll hold my breath if you don't buy me that."

Both Larry and Patrick had a similar body metabolism which lent itself to loss of consciousness from breath holding. Larry's mother was sensible and experienced and she had a warm, loving relationship with her son. She was justifiably concerned at first and sought medical help, but she was able to keep the breath-holding spells in perspective once she was reassured. Patrick had already dominated his mother by the time the initial breath-holding attack occurred. Because of inexperience, anxiety, and a poor mother-child relationship, an insignificant problem had been allowed to grow into a major behavioral difficulty. Treatment for Patrick and his mother consisted of a long period of counseling at a child guidance clinic after a thorough medical checkup and reassurance that the episodes themselves were not harmful.

The most satisfactory immediate treatment for a breath-holding spell, whether it is the first one or a repeat episode, is a sharp forceful slap on the buttocks. This accomplishes two things. It sets up a reflex which makes the child breathe, and it provides a genuinely unpleasant sensation to the child. Secondary treatment by the physician involves finding out whether the spell was coincidental or deliberate, the nature of the provoking circumstances, and counseling the family to be sure the child is neither punished nor rewarded as a result of the episode.

Some physicians have reported a high incidence of anemia from lack of iron in the diet in children who are subject to breath-holding. Theoretically an anemic child is more likely to pass out from lack of oxygen than one who is not anemic. There is some question about whether the incidence of anemia, common in the preschool age group, is coincidental. However, any child with several episodes of loss of consciousness following breath-holding deserves a thorough medical check-up, including a blood count. If the child's very brief episode of unconsciousness is characterized by repeated jerking movements, an EEG might be helpful in differentiating it from a true seizure.

Sometimes, an anatomical abnormality of the large blood vessels connected to the heart can cause brief periods of unconsciousness, which can be mistaken for seizures, in a very young infant. The abnormal blood vessel compresses the windpipe. If the area of compression is irritated by swallowing or coughing, a reflex causes breathing to stop. Infants with this condition have difficulty in swallowing, chest congestion, wheezing, and a peculiar brassy cough likened to a seal's bark. Treatment usually involves surgical correction of the abnormality.

**80
"Seal bark"
in young
infants**

This type of jerking movement occurs mainly in infants although it has been seen in children as old as 15 years. The child's head jerks slowly and irregularly, either up and down or from side to side. Most of the affected babies also have irregular eye movements and some will hold their heads at a particular angle in order to focus their vision. No cause is known. The condition often begins in the wintertime and is supposedly seen in children who spend a lot of time in dimly lit rooms. The condition will cure itself in several months and no treatment is necessary except for being sure that the baby gets enough light and air and a well-balanced diet with added vitamins.

**81
Nodding
spasms**

These are usually short, stereotyped movements unassociated with loss of consciousness. They can usually be interrupted by the voice (the victim's own or someone else's) or by the interference of another person. In most instances, the habit spasm is a mechanism for the release of tension and may be controlled by the child by concentration. For example, a child whose tic consists of stretching his neck may be able to control the movement as long as he thinks he is under observation. As soon as the period of observation is over and he seems to relax, the movement may occur several times in quick succession. Occasionally, an individual consciously or unconsciously learns a complicated series of movements or thoughts

**82
Tic or habit
spasm**

in order to prevent the tic from occurring. This is self-defeating—the new series of movements is also a tic. He may also learn how to stop a tic by grunting or swearing. In an advanced form, known as the tic of "Gilles de la Tourette," the series of movements, which are almost always performed in the same way, may last over a minute to complete and may end with an obscene remark. At first the remarks are made quietly or in private. As the movement disorder becomes more frequent, the accompanying obscenity is apt to be said loudly and in public.

Common tics are eye blinking, facial twitching, sniffling, and coughing. The term "habit spasm" is used when the movement is unconscious and almost beyond the control of the individual. Fatigue or unusual emotional stress will often bring on a tic. Treatment can vary from a simple search for stress in the child's environment to intensive psychotherapy. Certain drugs have also been found useful (for example, haloperidol).

MEDICAL TREATMENT
OF SEIZURES

The successful care of a child with chronic convulsions involves, first and foremost, control of his symptoms. The symptoms can be controlled directly by specific drugs and indirectly by making sure the child's environment is the best that can be created for him. Different children respond to drugs in different ways, and sometimes a long period of trial and observation is needed to find out which is the best medication for any particular child. Adjustment of the dosage generally must be made as the child grows.

83
What is good control?
It may be worthwhile to discuss what I mean by the term *control*. Theoretically, a drug can be given in an amount sufficient to suppress all seizures. This may not be desirable, how-

ever. The amount necessary to eliminate all seizures may produce serious side-effects such as drowsiness. If the primary aim is to eliminate seizures, rather than to control them, the child and his family tend to view each seizure as a catastrophe. It is much more reasonable to assume that an occasional spell may occur. The child and his family should look upon the period between the spells as being much more important than the spells themselves.

Up to five seizures a year can be considered evidence of good control provided they do not interfere with the child's activity at home or at school. If the medication can be increased without producing side-effects, it might be advisable to do so, so as to further limit the number of seizures. The early side-effects of overmedication may be mild and may develop gradually in children. The most common are increasing clumsiness and sleepiness. The child is often unable to describe vague symptoms. If a child takes one of the drugs which may affect the blood [90, 91], periodic blood counts are needed. Many of the serious side-effects of a drug are evident soon after the drug is started because the child has an *idiosyncrasy* (or unusual reaction) to that particular drug rather than because of an overdose.

DRUGS

The child with seizures, just as every other child, must become as independent and self-sufficient as he can. It is important to arrange a schedule which will allow the child to be responsible for his own medication. For example, one week's supply of medication can be left by the child's toothbrush. The routine of brushing the teeth twice a day and taking the medicine twice a day becomes a habit. A mother should not need to repeat the nagging question, "Did you take your medicine?" The drug should not be left on the dining table with the vitamins so that guests, relatives, brothers, and sisters are constantly reminded of the child's spells. The child should not become dependent on a parent to remind him to take the drug if he is capable of remembering it himself.

Administration of a drug in a liquid form (elixir of phenobarbital, for example), is much more expensive and far

84
How should
the drug
be given?

less accurate than giving the same drug as a tablet. The liquid can be easily spilled; a standard measuring spoon must be used, *and the parent must measure the dose.* Even a small infant can be given a tablet crushed in a small amount of honey or corn syrup. The use of suspensions of Dilantin is not desirable with children because the measurement of the drug in this form is too difficult. Even if a dropper is used and the bottle is shaken, mistakes occur.

85
What should I do if my child forgets a dose? It may happen rarely that a dose is omitted through accident or forgetfulness. The dose or doses omitted should be added to and given with the next scheduled dose. However, the total amount given in any 24-hour period should never exceed the total daily dose.

Drugs commonly used in the treatment of spells are discussed in the following sections. It may be helpful to parents and others to know what drugs are available, how they are used, and what side effects they may produce. *This section is not intended as a do-it-yourself guide for medication.* Each child will react to medication in an individual way, and it may take time before the physician works out the right combination.

86
Phenobarbital In the pediatric age group, this drug is undoubtedly the most useful for the management of most convulsive disorders. Phenobarbital is both a sedative and an anticonvulsant. Fortunately its sedative effect disappears after several days of use so that there is no interference with the child's sleeping patterns, learning ability, or behavior. The anticonvulsant effect builds up gradually in the body tissues until they become "saturated." It takes perhaps a week or ten days to achieve the anticonvulsant level and probably an equal amount of time to run out after the drug is stopped. This means that the drug will be effective if it is given twice a day and that the amount of the drug given today at 8 P.M. is equally as important in preventing a seizure as the amount that has been given regularly for the past two weeks. The drug should not be increased or decreased without a clear reason. For example, the easy thing for a parent to do is to give an extra dose of phenobarbital because the child is "active." Perhaps the

parent has from time to time taken phenobarbital himself for sedation and supposes the same result will occur in the child. *Phenobarbital is not a good drug for improving a child's behavior.* In fact, the use of any drug to affect behavior is a matter that *only* a physician can safely undertake.

There are occasional children who become hyperactive following the administration of phenobarbital. In most instances this occurs in children who have received small amounts or in whom there is considerable anxiety. A typical example of the "failure" of phenobarbital therapy is a three-year-old who is known to have febrile seizures who is given a phenobarbital tablet containing ¼ grain (15 mg). He continues to be very active and does not settle down to sleep. In this case, a true stimulating effect may be suspected by the physician. A more likely explanation, however, is that the purpose for which the medication was given or its dosage was not appropriate. This should not, however, exclude the possibility that it may be the best drug at some future time.

The amount of phenobarbital prescribed daily depends upon the weight of the child. Because the amount of the drug is measured in milligrams (mg), the traditional method of calculation is based upon the patient's weight in kilograms (kg). To find the weight in kilograms, the weight in pounds is divided by 2.2. The starting amount of 2–3 mg/kg per day is generally accepted until mid-adolescence. If more than 5–6 mg/kg is required for seizure control, it is generally preferable to add a second drug because long-term use of phenobarbital in large doses may be associated with undesirable side-effects. Discontinuation should be on a gradual basis since abrupt stoppage may precipitate the onset of frequent seizures. One of the most frequent causes for status epilepticus (prolonged severe recurrent seizures [64]) is in an otherwise reasonably controlled individual, is "running out" of medication. Several days will generally elapse between the time the drug is withdrawn and the onset of the seizures. During this time the individual may feel very well and may wonder if the medication is necessary.

More than 20 mg/kg in less than one hour is likely to produce severe drowsiness and slow, labored breathing. Rash,

**87
Dosage of
phenobarbital**

hyperactivity, and idiosyncratic responses are rare. Periodic blood and urine examination should be done at appropriate intervals as they would be for any well child—usually at the time of school and camp examinations.

88
Diphenylhy-
dantoin
(Dilantin)
Diphenylhydantoin, often prescribed in the form of Dilantin, is one of the most effective for the treatment of grand mal seizures. Although it may be used alone, I prefer to prescribe it in combination with at least one other anticonvulsant medication. The dosage is again based on weight and divided into two daily amounts; it is best given in tablet or capsule form since the liquid suspension is difficult to give correctly [84].

Most children can take 8 mg/kg of the drug each day on a regular basis without serious side-effects. There is almost always slight swelling (hyperplasia) of the gums near the teeth if the drug is continued for a period of time. The amount of gum hyperplasia does not always reflect the amount of drug received. If the swelling becomes objectionable, the amount of drug can be reduced by one-third. Good dental hygiene can often make the difference between successful control and something that is less than satisfactory. Use of an electric toothbrush often improves mouth care surprisingly.

In some instances, the measurement of the amount of diphenylhydantoin and other drugs in the blood serum is helpful. This is particularly desirable if more than one drug is being used and side-effects have occurred. Analysis by means of gas chromatography, if it is available, allows a rapid answer to the question of whether diphenylhydantoin or other drugs are found in the serum at their proper levels.

Less common side-effects of the drug include skin rash, dizziness, and blood abnormalities. Fortunately, idiosyncratic reactions are rare, but more than 12–15 mg/kg per day is generally not tolerated. In my experience, most side-effects have occurred following the use of the suspension, where an overdose is more likely than an unusual individual reaction. Reaction to an overdose of diphenylhydantoin should not lead to abrupt withdrawal. If this is done, the child may be deprived of the drug which would actually be the most effective for him if it were given in the right amounts. If an idiosyncratic response *has* occurred (that is, a drug reaction at low dosage—

especially shortly after it has been started), the drug should be withdrawn and not given again.

The administration of this drug for behavioral difficulties without definite seizures has been suggested. The evidence for the success of this treatment of children is not convincing, but some children who have "seizure equivalents" see [73, 74] could possibly benefit. Electroencephalography should help to identify these children.

Mebaral is chemically similar to phenobarbital and is some-times used if phenobarbital is not well tolerated. The dose is approximately twice that recommended for phenobarbital.

89 Mebaral (mepho-barbital)

Tridione is an effective drug in the treatment of *petit mal* seizures [67]. The recommended starting dose is 25 mg/kg per day in two to four doses. The physician may increase this dosage up to a maximum of 80 mg/kg per day in slow stages if necessary.

90 Tridione (trime-thadione)

However, Tridione used by itself may increase the pos-sibility of having *grand mal* attacks if the child is also susceptible to these seizures, and phenobarbital or Dilantin often have to be added. Tridione is one of the anticonvulsant drugs which can affect the blood, and periodic blood counts should be obtained if the drug is given for any length of time. Tridione may also cause nausea, drowsiness, and skin rashes. These symptoms disappear when the drug is discontinued. Because Tridione can harm the blood and kidneys, it has been replaced by Zarontin and other medications in most instances.

Zarontin has largely replaced Tridione as the most useful drug for the management of uncomplicated petit mal spells. Al-though some side-effects such as nausea, drowsiness, hic-coughing, and skin rash can appear, these symptoms usually disappear if the amount of medication is decreased. They usually do not recur if the drug is then restarted, increased more gradually and maintained below the previous level. Al-though it is very unusual for Zarontin to affect the blood, periodic blood counts should be obtained. The recommended starting dose is one capsule (250 mg) daily for a week. If necessary, the number of capsules given daily is increased by

91 Zarontin (ethosuxa-mide)

one each week until a total of six capsules a day is reached (two capsules, three times daily). A young child may be given the contents of the capsule mixed into an ounce of juice or of water with artificial sweetener added.

Most physicians nevertheless prefer to give a child who has petit mal seizures a trial of phenobarbital. Phenobarbital has fewer side effects, it is easier to give, and it is much cheaper. If phenobarbital alone does not control the spells, Zarontin is a good drug to add.

92
Mysoline
(primidone)

Mysoline is useful in the management of grand mal and psychomotor seizures. It is sometimes used in combination with other drugs. The chief side effects, such as drowsiness and skin rash, can usually be avoided by starting with small amounts (125 mg) at bedtime and increasing the dose very gradually at 7-to-10 day intervals to a maximum dose of 250 mg three times a day, for a total dose of 750 mg/day.

93
Valium
(diazepam)

Valium is a relatively new drug which looks promising in the management of infantile myoclonic seizures and petit mal spells which have not responded to other medication. Valium is also often given intravenously in a hospital to control status epilepticus when other, more conventional measures fail [64].

94
Tegretol
(carbama-
zepine)

Although its various side-effects have limited the use of this drug, it is often helpful. Reports from Europe concerning its use are encouraging, especially for children who have both petit mal and grand mal seizures.

NON-DRUG CONTROL

95
The
ketogenic
diet

It has been known for a long time that fasting, limitation of water intake and administration of certain types of foods will alter the body's chemical processes in such a way as to have an anticonvulsant effect (ketosis). This regimen is known as the *ketogenic diet*, and it was once commonly used for the management of petit mal and grand mal spells. There are many practical limitations to its use. The diet is unpalatable and rigid

—strict adherence can be quite a strain for both parents and children. The child is conspicuous in his family and in his group because of the special diet; it becomes almost impossible for him to feel that he is "normal" in spite of his seizures. The emotional problems caused by the diet far outweigh any dubious therapeutic advantages. Since its introduction over thirty years ago, the development of new and safe anticonvulsant drugs have limited its use. Ketosis can also be produced by a diet containing medium-chain triglycerides (MCT). While this diet is also difficult to maintain, it is better tolerated and more palatable.

CONDITIONS WHICH MAY BE ASSOCIATED WITH CONVULSIONS

Many children who have seizures have the idiopathic variety: After diligent search, no cause for the spells can be found. Management of the problem consists of bringing the seizures under control and helping the child and his family adjust their attitudes to insure a normal life. This generally presents no insurmountable problems because most youngsters with idiopathic seizures have normal intelligence and normal development. There are many handicapping conditions, however, which are often associated with seizures. In dealing with this type of problem one's perspective must change a little. The best possible management of the basic condition must be made the primary goal, rather than the totally successful treatment of the seizures. To be sure, the seizures must be controlled as far as possible, but both parents and physicians must realize that they are only part of the problem and that successful control of the convulsions will not specifically improve the underlying causes of the spells. There is a two-way relationship: Good control of the seizures will certainly

96
A
perspective

simplify the management of the basic condition; the best possible management of the basic condition will certainly help the seizures, for emotional stress and physical stress have an adverse effect on any convulsive disorder.

CEREBRAL PALSY

97
What is cerebral palsy?
The term *cerebral palsy* is used to describe a motor handicap of central origin. (*Motor handicap* means that the child cannot use his voluntary muscles as well as would be expected of someone his mental age; the term *central origin* means that the cause for this motor handicap lies in the brain rather than in the spinal cord or in the muscles.) There are many causes for cerebral palsy: premature birth, difficulties at birth, severe central nervous system infections, and head injuries are some of them. Not all premature births result in cerebral palsy, of course, and there may be no medical problems whatsoever following many head injuries, but these are common causes. A child may have cerebral palsy for no known reason. Convulsions may or may not be associated with cerebral palsy and a child with cerebral palsy may or may not be retarded.

At one time it was important to distinguish between cerebral palsy and poliomyelitis for administrative reasons. (Poliomyelitis may cause a motor handicap because of damage to the spinal cord rather than the brain.) Funds were available for treatment with polio. Now that immunization has made polio a rare disease in the United States, funds are more available for children with cerebral palsy. Currently it is easier to find funds for treatment for a child with convulsions and cerebral palsy than it is for a child who has convulsions and mental retardation (but not cerebral palsy) although the mental abilities of the two children may be identical.

98
Are there different kinds of cerebral palsy?
The common types of cerebral palsy are easy to identify. For example a child who has weakness of his right arm and right leg, without weakness in the facial muscles probably has congenital spastic hemiplegia. Many mild cases may not be recognized until the child begins to walk. Some of these children have abnormal EEGs [52], and they may have recurrent

seizures. The gradual development of symptoms in congenital spastic hemiplegia contrasts sharply with the rather sudden onset of a one-sided paralysis in a previously well child following a severe febrile illness with convulsions (such as in meningitis).

A second form of cerebral palsy is called spastic diplegia, or Little's disease; convulsions occur less commonly than in children with hemiplegia. The associated findings are a history of prematurity (birth weight of less than 5½ pounds), crossed eyes, and a tendency for the baby or child to "scissor" the legs and stand on the toes when he is held upright.

A third type, athetoid cerebral palsy, is unlikely to have seizures. Affected children have excessive and seemingly purposeless movements, caused by an injury to a particular part of the brain, the *basal ganglia*. A severe kind of infant-mother Rh incompatibility associated with jaundice is one cause of damage to the brain.

A fourth type, spastic quadriplegia, is frequently associated with convulsions and mental retardation. All four extremities are involved and the circumference of the head (and therefore the brain itself) tends to be small. Recurrent convulsions are common, but are a small part of the overall problem [147–151].

MENTAL RETARDATION

Although many children with mental retardation have convulsions, convulsions very rarely *cause* mental retardation. Whatever caused the child's mental retardation is usually also the cause of the convulsions.

Sometimes the assignment of a label such as "retarded trainable" is actually a handicap because it tends to cause people who work with a child never to *expect* him to do any better. This often means that the child is never given the opportunity to develop his full potential and, therefore, does not. In an excellent and progressive state training school in New England, teacher aides in training are purposely denied any medical information about a child's intellectual level—they approach the child as if there were no limit to his ability, and

99
Mental
retardation
and
convulsions

they patiently find out each child's limitations without a preconceived idea of what he can and cannot do.

Some background discussion concerning growth and
development may be helpful in understanding mental retardation. The standard tests or measurements compare a child's
performance or size against a "curve" of average children of
similar age and background. There is no average or normal
child. For example, if ninety-nine "normal" six-year-old boys
were ranked according to height, the third boy would be 42.7
inches tall; the middle or fiftieth boy, 46.3 inches tall; and the
97th, 49.7 inches. There would still be the first and second
boys who would be smaller than 42.7 inches and the 98th and
99th boys who would be taller than 49.7 inches. These four
boys are all the same age, physically well, and all are "normal." Other measures could be made of these 99 normal boys.
These could include weight (38.5 lb to 61.1 lb), head circumference, and other measurements of physical growth. Various
skills can also be defined. These include language use, social
age, and ability to solve problems requiring reasoning. The
children taken from the so-called normal population will
change position in the rank from 1 to 99, depending upon
what is being measured, so that the same child will rarely
be number 50 in each characteristic. If 97 out of 99 can do a
particular task or meet a certain standard, then it is customary
to say this is "normal."

The normal six-year-old will be over 42.7 inches tall,
weigh over 38.5 lb, be able to recognize 3 colors, put on his
coat, draw a recognizable man, take himself to the bathroom,
and sit in a chair when asked to do so.

When it is asked whether a child with a seizure disorder
is mentally or physically retarded, the answer can rarely be a
simple yes or no. An approximate answer can be given at that
point in time, but it is usually far more important to know how
fast the child learns or what his progress in acquiring new
skills may be. For this reason, it becomes highly desirable to
give the child as close to normal experience and activity as
possible.

For example, a child may not be able to draw a recognizable man only because he has not been allowed to hold a
crayon in his hand. This can have occurred innocently, because

the child has a tendency to put objects in his mouth, and his mother fears that he may have a convulsion and choke. The failure may then be the result of lack of experience. By itself failure to use a crayon may seem trivial, but if this kind of restriction is one of many, the child's development may have been unfavorably affected by attitudes toward him rather than by damage from the seizures themselves.

In recent years it has become fashionable to classify degrees of mental retardation by the child's IQ [26]. Children with IQ scores ranging from 90 to 110 are considered *normal;* those with scores from 80–90 are *low average* or *dull normal;* those whose IQs are in the 70–80 range are classified *borderline normal.* The borderline normal children are educable at a slower pace, and although they are not retarded, they find it hard to keep up in a regular class. They may be self-supporting in a somewhat protected community. In fact, even children in the dull normal category may have difficulties in highly competitive schools. Levels of retardation are classified by IQ scores obtained on various psychological tests [34–36]. According to a specific IQ score, a child's retardation could be classified as mild, moderate, severe, or profound. This rather arbitrary classification is useful from an administrative standpoint, but it does not really help (and may harm) an individual child. It is important to determine *what the child can do, not how "retarded" he is.*

100
What is mental retardation?

A child's achievement is, of course, influenced by his basic mental ability; it is also influenced by physical handicaps, social or emotional deprivation, family expectations, personality, appearance, and ability to get along with others. Chronic seizures could certainly hinder a child's achievement, however limited, if they were allowed to interfere with needed opportunities for development. A mother might not allow her child to climb stairs unassisted because she is afraid that he might have a convulsion and injure himself by falling down. This limitation is unrealistic and in itself is a far greater handicap than the convulsive disorder itself.

Educational facilities for retarded children vary widely according to the number of retarded children identified in the community, the funds available, and the experience of the personnel. A child with an IQ of 79 might get along very well in the regular class of a small elementary school in a rural community. He would not therefore be considered retarded in his particular environment. Another child with an IQ of 79 would be unable to keep up with the regular class of a big city school and would do much better in a "retarded educable" class. In his particular environment he is considered retarded. Each school administrative district sets up specific guidelines for educational classification of retarded children. These classifications vary greatly from district to district and there may be considerable flexibility within the individual community. In general, children with IQs between 50 and 70 are eligible for the *retarded trainable* classes and those with IQs from 30 to 49 are considered trainable, but there are few definite educational facilities for them and their training is carried out largely in private or community agency settings. Any child with an IQ below 29 is considered to need not formal education but rather *supportive care*. [This classification is that recommended by The American Association on Mental Deficiency.]

OTHER PROBLEMS

101 Cerebral dysfunction (learning disability, brain-injury) George, a nine-year-old boy, was brought to the diagnostic center by his parents because of their increasing concern with his poor school performance. Although George was repeating second grade, he was reading only at first grade level. He could not cope with any kind of arithmetical reasoning, and his handwriting was virtually illegible. His teacher noted that he was easily distracted and that he was very restless in class. He would often get up from his desk, knocking over chairs and books in the process. He seemed to have a good memory for facts and details, and he enjoyed work in social studies and science if he did not have to read or write. He was something of a clown in class, and he enjoyed getting attention.

At home he occasionally had temper tantrums when attempts were made to discipline him. Although he was generally clumsy, he could ride a bicycle with some skill. His mother was apprehensive about his riding in the street because he was impulsive and he seemed to lack sound judgment. He enjoyed television and his family allowed him to watch a great deal. It seemed to be a "safe" activity.

George was the only boy in his family and the middle child. His sisters were twelve and five. He had been a little slow walking and talking, but not enough to cause any real concern. At the age of five he had had the first of three short grand mal seizures. He had a borderline abnormal EEG and the seizures were diagnosed as being idiopathic in origin. He had been seizure-free for three years after starting on a small daily dose of phenobarbital. There was no history of serious illness or accident. His birth history was considered normal.

Neurological examination showed that George confused his right and his left easily; he had difficulty with tests for balance. Psychological testing revealed that he had a normal full scale IQ of 95, but his verbal score was far ahead of his performance score [34]. He showed a great deal of scatter in his test results. He could not reproduce drawings; he often copied them backward, and he had great difficulty in separating an object from its background.

His parents were convinced that he could do good school work if "he would only pay attention," but they conceded that he was a disciplinary problem. They wondered if his learning difficulties were related to his convulsions in some way.

The terms *cerebral dysfunction, the hyperkinetic child, the brain-injured child,* and *the child with learning disability* could all be used to describe George's symptoms. He had normal intelligence, but perceptual difficulties and difficulties in abstract reasoning impeded his progress in school. He could learn, but he went about it in ways different from most other children. Children like George are often, but not always, hyperactive, clumsy, and emotionally volatile. Their problems are compounded by mounting frustration, when they are put into a learning situation in which they cannot succeed. Although they try hard, they find only failure and increasing parental and teacher exasperation. Many children with cerebral dysfunction have abnormal EEGs or a history of a convulsive disorder—many do not. There is no known cause-and-effect relationship, but the family's concern about his convulsions may spill over and complicate their feelings about the school failure.

102
What causes cerebral dysfunction?

The term *cerebral dysfunction* and the others used synonymously with it are purely descriptive and apply to a group of symptoms. Sometimes there is a known history of injury to the brain, caused by difficulties during birth, by accident (such as near-drowning), by infection (such as encephalitis), or by poison such as lead. There is often no known history of injury to the brain. Theoretically, this means either that the brain cells were injured in some obscure way at some particular point in time or that there has been some interference in the functional organization of the brain. The injury is more subtle than the kind which would produce cerebral palsy. (See glossary: brain damage).

But this theory of brain injury is really too simple. Many children have specific learning disabilities in certain areas such as reading, but they have none of the other symptoms described above. A child may have a serious central nervous system infection or a period of prolonged unconsciousness from an auto accident and have no residual symptoms whatsoever. Some children with learning problems caused by "brain injury" improve with time. Although the incidence of abnormal EEGs is higher in brain-injured children than in the population at large, there is no convincing evidence that a particular area of the brain is injured. The theory of a known or unknown subtle injury to the brain is attractive, but not proven. Cerebral dysfunction is, therefore, only a descriptive term.

103
What is the treatment for cerebral dysfunction?

Treatment is relatively simple and effective. Unfortunately, it is also both expensive and difficult to find. The first step is to create an atmosphere in which success is inevitable. A program may need to be created especially for the individual. Sometimes a teacher who has some skill and training in special education can apply special techniques directly. These may be an extension of the tests that the child succeeded in doing on his psychological examination. If the child's environment at home has placed too many pressures and conflicting ideas upon him, it may be difficult to reorient the attitudes of others toward him, and to reorient his own pessimistic attitude toward himself.

It is not unusual to find a child who has presumably "passed" third grade but who cannot read. A different method of teaching reading (phonic rather than whole-word, for example) may be needed. Instead of being discouraged, a skilled teacher can turn the situation into a positive one by showing the child that he can learn the same material in a different way. Once the child has been convinced that he is not a failure, a series of successes of increasing difficulty can be arranged for him.

Although the child may learn to work well in a group, the educational problem increases if the child is behind in more than one subject. By the very nature of special education, it is difficult for one teacher to have more than six to eight students. Groups of compatible children may be difficult to assemble. For these reasons, it is highly desirable to recognize learning disabilities early and to treat them promptly— delay makes them more difficult to solve. Obviously, management problems at home can create additional learning difficulties and make matters worse. In most instances, it is possible to keep the child in his regular class if the difficulty is recognized early and dealt with effectively.

Treatment with drugs, except for convulsions, is ineffective unless remedial work is both available and appropriate. Too often, psychic stimulating drugs (Benzidrine, Dexidrine, Ritalin), tranquilizing agents (Thorazine, Atarax, Vistaril) or sedatives (barbiturates) are substituted for a sound program of social, educational, and recreational habilitation [130, 137].

Children occasionally develop diseases which cause the central nervous system to lose the ability to function properly. Tay-Sachs disease is such a condition. There are several others. Although convulsions may occur early in the course of the illness, other symptoms are almost always present. Sometimes these symptoms are the gradual loss of abilities and skills which have already been learned. Most of these conditions are very rare and may be clearly identified only by examination of the brain itself. One way this can be done is the *cerebral*

104 Degenerative disease of the central nervous system

biopsy, a procedure which requires a neurosurgical operation to remove a small portion (usually less than a one-half inch square) from a "silent" or unused area of the brain. This kind of operation is usually restricted to those medical centers where rather sophisticated laboratory facilities are available. The procedure perhaps sounds more difficult than experience has shown it to be. This is one of the methods which may prove to be helpful in understanding the chemical and structural basis for diseases which do not have specific treatment.

The possibility of a degenerative disease should be suggested by gradual loss of motor, mental, visual, or language function over a period of weeks or months. Children develop skills in an orderly way, and once a skill such as walking is mastered, it is rarely lost without cause. A doctor would also be concerned about a child who failed to learn new skills at the expected time if his previous history up to that point has been normal.

For this reason, knowledge of his growth and development helps to identify at the earliest possible moment his failure to mature.

Each child who has a degenerative disease is unique. The physician will need to explain both the nature of the disease and how it affects the child. On the basis of his experience with other children who have been affected by similiar conditions, he will be able to answer most of the questions concerning problems of care and management. Even if the disease itself is not correctable, the physical care of the child can be maintained at a high level of professional competence.

BODY CHEMISTRY DISTURBANCES

Distortions in body chemistry may also cause convulsions. The exact biochemical reasons may not always be clear and treatment is usually directed toward the basic condition rather than toward the spells.

105 (PKU) Phenylketonuria (PKU) is a good example of an inherited basic disturbance in body chemistry which can cause convulsions. A child with PKU cannot absorb a certain part of protein (an amino acid, phenylalanine). The abnormally high blood levels of phenylalanine may in some way damage the brain, resulting in mental retardation and convulsions, usually of the minor motor [69] or petit mal [67] variety. Fortunately, a special low phenylalanine diet started very early in infancy can minimize the brain damage and eliminate the convulsions. Many states have laws requiring that each newborn baby be tested for PKU by means of a simple test using a drop of blood from the heel. If a baby suddenly begins to have petit mal or infantile myoclonic seizures the doctor will always check again for PKU or make sure that the baby has been adequately tested. The best results from the diet are obtained if the diet is started very early, but improvement nearly always occurs if the diet is started before two years of age.

105
Phenylketo-
nuria (PKU)
and other
"inborn
errors of
metabolism"

Another example of an inherited amino acid disorder which can cause convulsions is Maple Syrup Urine Disease, so named because of the characteristic odor of the urine. A special rigid diet low in certain amino acids is believed to help prevent mental damage if the diagnosis is made during the first few weeks of life. Unfortunately, dietary treatment for this condition is still experimental.

Seizures are a rare symptom of Wilson's Disease, an uncommon inherited disorder of copper metabolism. Early and prolonged administration of a diet high in protein and low in copper is helpful.

Low blood sugar can be associated with an alarming change in consciousness; recurrent loss of consciousness from low blood sugar is sometimes preceded by personality and behavioral changes.

106
Low blood
sugar (hypo-
glycemia)

The cause of low blood sugar in young children is poorly understood. If the blood sugar level is consistently found to be low, treatment with an appropriate drug (usually related to cortisone) may relieve the symptoms and raise the blood sugar to more normal levels. However, the blood sugar of some babies may go down just with normal feeding. Such infants are generally found to be sensitive to an amino acid, called leucine, found in milk. A special diet may help correct this difficulty. As the child grows older and milk becomes a less important part of his normal diet, leucine sensitivity becomes less apparent.

The blood sugar of some children is normal between

episodes of loss of consciousness, making it difficult to confirm a diagnosis of hypoglycemia. It may be normal after an overnight fast. Because of its sporadic nature, even more complicated tests lasting 5 or 6 hours may yield only normal levels, even in children who do have low blood sugar levels (less than 35 mg glucose/100 ml blood) at the time of an episode [57].

When certain substances called ketones are present in the urine of hypoglycemic children, the term *ketotic hypoglycemia* has been used. This condition usually clears up spontaneously after 7 or 8 years of age and is rare before 2 years. Treatment consists of feeding at night before sleep and the prompt administration of orange juice (which contains sugar) within 15 minutes after awaking to prevent episodes of unconsciousness from occurring. The episode itself can be ended by giving sugar by mouth. An intravenous injection (given in the hospital) might be necessary if the child cannot swallow. The administration of glucagon, a compound which may be helpful in patients with low blood sugar associated with diabetes, is often ineffective in this condition.

107 Kidney disease One of the complications of severe kidney disease is the development of high blood pressure. Sometimes the high blood pressure causes a narrowing of the blood vessels in the brain—headache, vomiting, drowsiness, and convulsions result. Treatment, of course, is aimed at reducing the high blood pressure. Sometimes anticonvulsants, such as phenobarbital and Dilantin, need to be added.

108 Tetany *Tetany* is a term used to describe increased irritability of the muscles and nerves. Certain distortions in some chemical compounds of the body, such as calcium, produce this state. If the distortion is great enough, actual convulsions may result. The treatment is based on correcting the body chemistry rather than on the administration of an anticonvulsant drug.

109 Lead poisoning There is an old wives' tale that children who are allowed to chew on combs will have fits. This bit of folklore was true until manufacturers stopped making combs out of lead, but lead poisoning is still relatively common. Lead builds up in the body over a period of time and can cause swelling of the brain and convulsions. Lead poisoning can cause permanent brain damage, and a child may continue to have spells long after the acute phase of his illness has passed. Convulsions from lead poisoning can be prevented, of course. Children should not be allowed to chew old paint and plaster, and toys, cribs, and furniture should all be painted with nontoxic compounds.

PART THREE

The Environment

YOUR CHILD'S WORLD

In the two preceding sections, I have discussed the background and the medical management of seizures. Some of the information has been factual, some of it has been theoretical. Most of it concerned scientific matters, namely the diagnosis and treatment of seizures. If a convulsive disorder had a beginning, an end, an inevitably identifiable cause, and an infallible treatment, this book could end right here. Unfortunately, this is not the case. Seizures are not like measles. Sometimes the beginning is indefinite, the cause is obscure, the treatment is merely promising and the end may not be in sight.

Ignorance and despair breed suspicion and prejudice. Convulsive disorders have been with mankind for a long time, and a climate of misunderstanding has arisen over the centuries. During the past thirty-five years, great advances have been made in the treatment of epilepsy and in the treatment of some of the medical conditions of which recurrent seizures may be a part. Many of the old, restrictive laws passed in bygone days of ignorance and superstition have been amended or repealed. In spite of this progress, however, any affected child and/or family is going to come into contact with a negative reaction at some point. For example, there is a widespread notion that chronic seizures somehow predispose the individual to commit a crime. Occasionally a person accused of a crime of violence receives nationwide publicity when it is brought out that he has an abnormal EEG. There is no convincing evidence of a connection between the EEG and the aberrant behavior. Most people with abnormal EEGs are not criminals, and many people with normal EEGs commit crimes. That a crime of passion could be committed by an otherwise responsible person during a seizure-induced "dream" state is highly speculative and probably a myth.

If a positive environment can be created for the child in the home, the school, and the community, he will hopefully be able to develop a sound outlook which will enable him to cope with any difficulties he may encounter. The creation of this environment is a major part of the successful treatment of a convulsive disorder. That is what this section of the book is all about.

THE PARENTS' ROLE

**110
How can my
attitudes
affect
my child?** The parents' attitudes toward their child will determine in a major way the child's attitude toward himself. He will develop confidence in himself if those around him have confidence in him. Although associated medical handicaps might predispose him to various types of illness or injury, a child with seizures usually will have the same number of colds, stomachaches, bruises, and injuries as his brothers and sisters. He seems to be different primarily because the adults around him over-respond to any complaint he may have. This fear that he may have a seizure may be more crippling than the seizure itself. They *expect* him to respond differently, and he does.

First of all, the parents must consider themselves competent. They should develop the feeling that they are doing as well as they, or anyone else, could do under the circumstances. Their feelings of guilt, despair, or hostility may be readily sensed by the child and may make matters worse. Some parents may be overwhelmed at first by the problems presented by a child with chronic seizures. It takes time to develop feelings of competence and to reduce or eliminate feelings of guilt. Professional help may be needed to clarify matters [149].

A sound parent-physician relationship is basic to the development of an appropriate attitude toward the child. The parents must have complete confidence in their physician over a period of time. They must feel that the management of their child's condition is in the best of hands. Quick cures and pat answers are never found in the management of recurrent seizures.

Sometimes, parents or well-meaning relatives become convinced that one single approach such as a tonsillectomy will stop the convulsions once and for all. The pressure on the doctor can be almost intolerable. The wise physician will point out that the tonsils are not causing the seizures and that tonsillectomy has complications of its own. He will also bring up a much more important fact: The disappointment and frustration felt by the family when their hopes are dashed and the magic cure doesn't work can cause serious psychological damage to the parents as well as the child. The physician should also be alert to the parents' needs. Some mothers need to be reassured constantly; some are competent and well informed; some cover a basic insecurity with a facade of competence. The astute physician can sort these out and help each in the most appropriate fashion.

Finally, the parents must keep informed about their child's condition and about convulsive seizures in general. They will be asked many questions by family, friends, and the community. If they are up-to-date and knowledgeable they can set errors in thinking right and perhaps in a small way improve the climate of opinion around them.

111 How should I discipline my child?

He should be treated normally as far as his capabilities allow. He should not be punished for not doing something he is unable to do, but no excuses should be made for bad behavior because "he has seizures." The other children in the family will be quick to sense preferential treatment. In addition, almost any child will recognize and capitalize upon a situation that allows him to control or manipulate his parents. Fair play in the application of the family standards of discipline is vital.

112 Why some parents cannot manage the child with seizures.

Many parents who have no trouble in managing their other children change their attitudes and react differently to the actions and manner of the child with seizures. No single answer or explanation is satisfactory. Difficulty could occur under the following circumstances: (1) The parents see the child as being more vulnerable; (2) They overprotect him, often without realizing it; (3) They become overly concerned about how they are bringing up the child ("Am I doing the right thing?"); (4) The child feels insecure; (5) The child fails to understand what his parents expect of him.

These circumstances can cause the parents to become inconsistent, confused, and lose confidence in their ability to control the child. Because their reactions are not spontaneous, they contribute to or increase the child's feeling of insecurity. The child responds by teasing, tantalizing, and testing his limits. For example, a child with seizures may want to watch a program on television. If he is not allowed to do what he wants, he has a tantrum. His parents believe that his tantrum will lead to a seizure. If they mistakenly believe a seizure will cause permanent brain damage or that he will die during the seizure, they "give in." The result may be chaotic if this kind of pattern persists and may lead to the parents being unable to manage the child effectively. Professional guidance may be needed to improve matters [149].

SPORTS

113 Should his activities be limited in any way? There is no clear answer to what activities should be limited. It depends on many things. What kind of spells does he have? When is he likely to have them? Is he well coordinated? Does he have good judgment? The first question to ask oneself is, "Is the activity appropriate for a child of his age and ability who does not have spells?" The next question is, "Can he do it?" For example, should a four-year-old girl with grand mal seizures under good control be allowed to use a plastic wading pool in the backyard? The answer: of course, provided someone is with her. No four-year-old should use a plastic wading pool unsupervised. *The restriction is based on common sense, not the presence or absence of seizures.*

114 Should he ride a bicycle? The answer to this question again depends on the child. If he is a reasonably well-coordinated three- or four-year-old whose seizures are under good control he certainly can ride a tricycle in the backyard. Whether or not he can ride on the sidewalk depends on the neighborhood, the traffic, and on his temperament. A sensible ten-year-old who has spells only at night can be trusted with a two-wheeler. A reckless, impulsive eleven-year-old who has an occasional spell during the afternoon cannot. A reckless, impulsive, poorly coordinated eleven-year-old with no spells at all should not be trusted on a bicycle in the street either, however.

Even more variables must be considered in answering this question. Where will the riding take place? Will it be in a ring, on a bridle path, or on a mountain trail? How spirited is the horse? How skillful a rider is the child? Most children, and indeed most adults, fall off horses occasionally. There is therefore an added risk of injury. The anxiety centered about the injury may be more dangerous than the injury itself. How much does riding mean to the child? If the family gives an arbitrary "no" to the request, the child may suddenly decide horseback riding is the one thing he wants to do more than anything else.

**115
What about
horseback
riding?**

Swimming is an excellent sport. The child should be well supervised and if possible should receive instruction in water skills. Neither he nor anyone else should ever swim alone [77].

**116
Should my
child swim?**

Contact sports, like riding, provide more opportunity for injury. Is the sport worth it? If the answer is yes, the parent must be sure that the activity in question is properly supervised for a child of the same age and ability without spells. Most pediatricians disapprove of tackle football for the Junior High age group. Children of this age are in the midst of a growth spurt and young teenagers are particularly vulnerable to orthopedic injury. Are the teams well matched physically? Is there adequate coaching without adult exploitation of the youngsters' skills? Does the boy have the physical size and the athletic ability to make the team and get satisfaction from the activity? If the answers to these questions are yes, then he can go ahead, provided the seizures are under good control. Sometimes it is easier to channel an athletic youngster into tennis, golf, or track, thereby bypassing the need to prove himself by skill in football or soccer. Tennis can be started earlier, it can be played throughout life, and the satisfaction to the child is tremendous.

**117
Should he
play
football,
lacrosse,
or soccer?**

118
What about skiing?
A great deal would depend on the type of skiing and the skill of the youngster. How good a skier was he before the onset of seizures? How difficult are the slopes he plans to use? Is a chair lift necessary? When do his spells usually occur? What kind of spells are they? If the boy or girl skis very well, if the spells are under excellent control, and if skiing means the world to the child, the answer might be a very qualified yes. If a child has never been on skis I would see no reason to begin. Ice skating would be a far more appropriate activity.

THE CHILD'S RELATIONSHIP TO HIS WORLD

119
What should I tell my child about his condition?
The answer to this question is simple to write down but difficult to carry out. A parent should tell the child the truth. The truth told to a four-year-old is far less complicated than the truth told to a fourteen-year-old. The child should be told the facts with the amount of detail appropriate for his age and understanding. The emphasis should be that the spells are a *medical* condition for which medication is given. A four-year-old might be told "once long ago you were very sick. You were given medicine and got all better but a little of that sickness stayed with you and used to make you have sort of dizzy spells. Maybe the day will come when you won't have to take any pills at all." If there is no known cause for the spells, the child might be told that some people have "dizzy" spells for some reason and that pills prevent most of them.

A teenager will, of course, want a much more detailed explanation and he will need to be reassured that he will be able to do most things within his capabilities. He may ask if he has epilepsy. Since epilepsy means simply a convulsive disorder which is recurrent, it might seem that a simple yes would suffice. Unfortunately, however, many people associate the word with vague ideas of degenerative disease and insanity. That, of course, is completely false, but because of this long-standing negative attitude, I find it better to avoid the use of the word unless it has been clearly defined and understood. I would say to the inquiring teenager, "Yes, you have epilepsy, but let's discuss what it means. A lot of people have the wrong idea about it."

In general, the child should be present when the doctor talks to the parents, otherwise he will feel that there may be something mysterious and frightening about his condition. The parent who talks to the child about his spells must be well and accurately informed, and he must also be matter-of-fact and reassuring in his discussion. Sometimes a private talk between the child and his doctor can ease the communication gap.

Again, they should be told the truth. The child's brothers and sisters should have a fairly full explanation consistent with their age. If the explanation can be direct, reassuring, and positive they will transmit a positive attitude to the child who has the spells. He will be no more and no less than a member of the family who happens to have a medical problem.

120 What should I tell my family?

Sharing information with grandparents and older relatives can be difficult. Older people may have rather fixed ideas about medical matters, and their ideas about convulsions are not likely to be up-to-date. The tone and the manner in which the explanation is given are as important as the facts. In general, a good rule to remember is: the older the person, the fewer the facts.

The ideal parents have built up a solid positive attitude about the child's condition and have hopefully transmitted it to the child. This attitude will be essential in allowing the child to become a self-sufficient person.

Every child with or without spells must develop a feeling of competence and self-reliance. From the very earliest months he should be allowed and encouraged to develop as far as his capabilities will permit. It is natural for parents to overprotect a child with seizures. It is also natural for them to push him beyond his ability to prove he is normal. Either extreme can lead to difficult problems.

121 How can I help my child become independent?

The child who is never allowed to do things because he might get hurt grows up fearful and lacking in basic skills and self-confidence. The child pushed beyond his abilities may become withdrawn and he may refuse to attempt any new skill at home or at school because he fears failure. The parents must be realistic in their expectations. For example, most six-year-olds can tie their shoelaces, but it is not unusual for boys, especially, to be unable to master this rather complicated act before about seven years. If the parents make a big thing of tying shoelaces, six-year-old Johnny may feel he is failing them somehow by not learning to tie his shoes. Both he and his parents may wonder deep down if his spells have something to do with his failure. The simplest approach would be to forget the shoelaces for a while. Use cowboy boots or loafers and emphasize how well Johnny is doing in his swimming lessons.

Independence in taking medication should be encouraged as soon as possible. If the child takes his pill as naturally as he brushes his teeth, the fact that he has to take it loses a great deal of its threatening significance in his mind and in the minds of his parents.

**122
Responsi-
bility**

A child who is independent up to the limit of his ability should be encouraged to take on responsibility. This responsibility can range from the simplest household chores to caring for pets, baby-sitting, and doing jobs in the community such as delivering newspapers. A child may think to himself, "I have spells, so I'm different. There must be something really wrong with me. I'll never be any good." If he can be taught to assume responsibility his attitude may change to "I am an important person. I do this well. That's why they asked *me* to do it."

**123
What about
relationships
to his
playmates?**

A youngster whose convulsions began in very early childhood may have some difficulty in getting along with children his own age. The convulsions themselves are not the cause. The problem of attitude is again the culprit. If his mother has overprotected him, kept him close to her, and has not allowed him to develop independence and a positive attitude toward himself, he is going to be socially handicapped. Most children are remarkably matter-of-fact about medical conditions, and most are remarkably perceptive about the attitude of adults around them. If Jane's mother states the simple unvarnished truth, "Occasionally Jane has convulsions, but she's taking medicine for them and she hardly ever gets them now," Jane's friends will reply "So what?" and they will all troop out to play. If the mother had said, "Jane has convulsions, so you must be careful and not be too rough with her," the group would have looked uneasy and might have left without her.

Some children are social butterflies. Some are quiet. Some gather a gang of friends with no effort; others are more cautious in their approach to playmates. The presence of seizures should not alter the child's basic personality. If a vivacious, social mother happens to have a child who is quiet and who happens to have seizures, she should not make matters worse by blaming the seizures for his lack of social adaptability. This type of child might, however, benefit from a little outside help in developing social relationships, and this might best be done in some sort of supervised group activity such as a community recreation program or a day camp.

A keystone in child development is the search for identity—to find out, "What kind of a person am I?" This search comes to a head in adolescence. The young adult who has found himself, who knows who he is, what he is doing, and what he wants to do has found his identity. He has observed adults around him in his home, in his community, and in the world. Consciously or subconsciously he has formed his personality and ambitions after sorting out those traits he thinks are worthwhile. The child with seizures is so susceptible to a self-defeating, negative attitude toward himself that he desperately needs the presence of adults with whom he can identify. A boy needs a father or a father figure. A girl needs a mother. This is obvious. The attitude of the parents toward other adults in the child's world will also be a major factor in shaping his identity.

124
**The adults
in his world**

Bill's father constantly praises Bill's 21-year-old brother who was a three-letter man and honor student in high school. Bill has the impression that the most important goals in life are academic superiority and athletic stardom. He knows he is clumsy in sports and he is getting only average grades even though he tries hard. Bill feels he is a failure in life at the age of twelve.

Susan is all thumbs at sewing, and she always spills the milk and the flour when cooking. Her mother tells her constantly, "When I was your age I was making my own clothes and cooking dinner for six." Susan at thirteen feels that there is no hope for her.

The situation really gets complicated when the parents feel the convulsions may be the reason for their children's failure. This is not true, of course. Many honor students and athletes have spells, and so do many expert seamstresses and cooks. It would be much better to admire qualities which are actually possessed by the children or ones which are within their grasp. Praise from a camp counselor who is patient, persevering, and an expert woodsman might be more valuable for Bill. Susan might respond to the esteem in which a dedicated teacher is held in the community. The occupations of the model adults held up as examples to the child matter little. Their personalities, ways of life, and the strength of their own characters matter a great deal.

THE TEEN YEARS

125
The
adolescent

The adolescent with seizures really needs a solid self-image. Adolescence is a stormy time under the best of circumstances, and the pressure of a chronic medical condition usually tends to complicate matters. If the teenager has built up an inner feeling of competence during childhood, things will be much easier, whether he has had the spells for a long time or whether, as is common, the onset of the spells occurs during the teenage years.

Adolescents are intensely interested in their own maturing bodies. They will be likely to have some deep and sincere questions about their condition, and they will have some honest but strange misconceptions. Sometimes these are best answered in a private talk with the family doctor. To the usual adolescent question, "Who am I and where am I going?" must be added "What do these convulsions mean for me?"

The parents must be very clear in their own minds as to what part of their teenager's behavior, if any, is the direct result of the convulsive disorder. It is normal for any adolescent girl or boy to be selfish, moody, rebellious, and exasperating. It is also normal for them to be idealistic, creative, hard-working, and concerned. The convulsions themselves may have very little to do with their behavior—the attitude toward the spells has a great deal to do with their actions. Fortunately, both the attitude of their parents and their own attitude toward themselves can be helped to shift in a positive direction.

Sometimes adolescents will rebel against their parents by doing something likely to upset them. A thing sure to upset them is the omission of the daily anticonvulsant drug. The parent should be careful not to be drawn into a fight by over-reacting. This is exactly what the adolescent may want. The parents should point out the need for the drug in a matter-of-fact, nonthreatening way. The child doesn't really want the spell because it limits many activities—driving, for example [128]. A common-sense reaction from the parents may help him cool off. If a spell occurs because medication has been omitted, it should be handled in a routine manner without too much said about the cause. The parents might ask themselves what brought on the need to rebel? Is the parental rein too tight or too loose? Competent adolescents who have been responsible for their own medication for a period of years rarely rebel by omitting a dose [85]. Encouraging the teenager to deal directly with his doctor may be helpful.

**126
Rebellion over medication**

Any drug given for any reason can be abused by the person who takes it. However, teenagers on anticonvulsants are no more likely to experiment with "recreational" drugs than others of their age. Anticonvulsants are so much a part of their lives that drugs tend to lose attraction as a dubious source of illicit pleasure. Taking a pill is a chore rather than a thrill. A youngster who is already taking a maintenance dose of an anticonvulsant does not have any characteristic physical reaction to drug experimentation. If he feels the need to rebel he is much more likely to omit drugs rather than take them.

There is a rather widespread myth that seizures can be prevented by smoking marihuana. There is absolutely no evidence that this is true, and there seems to be no increase in its use among persons with convulsions. There is also no firm evidence that smoking marihuana is harmful to a youngster

**127
Is there danger of drug abuse from anti-convulsants?**

who has spells. However, because marihuana must be obtained illegally, its composition is uncertain. The individual's response is conditioned by the kind of response he expects to have, the actual chemical composition of the sample, his own physical reaction to drugs of any sort, and by any basic emotional problems already present.

Some persons have no subjective experience at all. The usual effect of marihuana is that of a pleasant, mild sedative. Unpleasant reactions include headache, nausea, and transient psychiatric disturbances.

Hallucinations usually occur only as a manifestation of toxic overdose. A marihuana user, with or without a previous history of seizures, may become acutely depressed, but more commonly he becomes anxious, tearful, and restless. He is able to relate his distress to consumption of the drug and respond to gentle authority. If the individual has taken other drugs which have produced hallucinations in the past, the experience may recur after smoking marihuana. Rarely, an individual may find that after a few minutes of pleasure, weird and unreal sensations occur which persist for several days. In these instances the intoxication with marihuana triggers an emotional problem, the basis of which already existed.

128
Driving
The big event for a boy or girl in mid-adolescence is the moment he or she gets a driver's license. Many youngsters with seizures must wait a little longer for that moment than they would if they did not have the spells. The age and the circumstances under which a person with seizures can legally drive vary widely from state to state. In my own state, Pennsylvania, a license may be issued to someone over sixteen who has been seizure-free for two years, with or without medication, and who presents a doctor's certificate to that effect. Sometimes a license may be granted to an individual in Pennsylvania after one year free from seizures if his spells occur only at night. Some people (for example, those with light-induced seizures) might be wise not to drive at all. The doctor and the family, of course, will consider whether the boy or girl is mature, responsible and coordinated enough to operate a motor vehicle even if he did not have convulsions. There is nothing magic about age sixteen. The skills necessary

to drive a car develop later in some people than in others. The need to be seizure-free for a long period of time can be an excellent incentive for remembering medication and taking good care of one's health.

Driver's licenses are now granted in all states to epileptics who supply satisfactory evidence that their seizures have been under control for a reasonable time and they can operate a car safely. Unfortunately, the regulations are not the same in each state. A condensed list of the state laws regarding issuance of driver's licenses is presented in Appendix 3.

Authorities in the state of Wisconsin pioneered in the establishment of reasonable regulations for issuance of driver's licenses to persons with controlled recurrent seizures. The Wisconsin statute provides that a temporary license, renewable every 6 months, may be issued by the Commissioner of Motor Vehicles if the applicant submits a special certificate from his physician stating that he is seizure-free and is competent to drive an automobile.

Ten years ago, few individuals with controlled seizures were granted driver's licenses. The last decade has proved that the driver whose seizures are under good control has an excellent safety record. He knows his license could be permanently revoked in case of an accident and he is likely to drive more carefully than the average driver.

EDUCATION

A major part of any child's total environment is, of course, school. The proper attitude toward the child and his problem on the part of teachers, school administrators, and fellow pupils can help a child achieve the ultimate goal of education. That goal is the same for him as it is for any child, namely the development of the child to his own highest capabilities in preparation for the work of life. How and where this is carried out depends on the resources of the child and also on the resources of the family and the community.

Children with seizures may have completely normal intelligence, or they may be retarded, or they may be physically handicapped, or they may be both retarded and handicapped.

No matter what associated difficulties they have, the fact that they have *seizures* singles them out immediately; it is almost as if they are marked "fragile, handle with care, use extreme caution, this side up." It would be much better if the child could be simply marked "rattle ok." Most teachers can handle difficult behavior problems or children with mental or motor handicaps with great competence. Yet, these very same teachers will suddenly feel helpless and tense when told that a particular child has seizures. This is all unnecessary, of course, but a climate of misunderstanding which has developed over hundreds of years dies hard. All teachers in all schools *should* be informed about convulsive disorders and enlightened about the proper approach to them, but many are not.

130
What kind of school is proper for my child?

The answer, of course, depends on the child and on the presence of any associated handicaps. The most important thing is to put the child in a school situation in which he will be successful. A child who has the onset of idiopathic seizures in late childhood and who is of normal intelligence will probably do perfectly well in a regular school. A child who has seizures and a reading disability might or might not do well in a regular school. It would depend on the type of remedial help available either within the school or within the community. A child who has seizures and whose mental ability is borderline would gain nothing by struggling in a regular class in a competitive, high-pressure school. In all likelihood, his all-important self-image would fail to develop, he would learn nothing, and he would make no progress. In an appropriate special class he would make progress, he could succeed, and his eagerness to learn would continue.

Sometimes just the physical qualities of the school are important. One ten-year-old girl hated school and made poor progress even though her intelligence was satisfactory and her grand mal seizures were well controlled. She had mild cerebral palsy and she was quite clumsy on her feet. It turned out that the bathroom in the seventy-five-year-old school was at the top of three flights of stairs. Her teacher was afraid she would have a convulsion and fall downstairs, so she always detailed another pupil to accompany her to the bathroom. The little girl could have managed the stairs alone if given a little extra time, but the fear felt by the teacher was transmitted to her and she became afraid to go alone. Because of her seizures she had been singled out and she became a target of ridicule. Transfer to a class with an enlightened teacher, in another school which was built on one level solved the problem.

In the final analysis the presence of seizures is not really important in the choice of school. The normal child, the retarded child, and the physically handicapped child must all be able to achieve success, and it is the ability of a school to provide the child with this opportunity that must be the primary consideration.

131 Is nursery school a good idea?

The very young child (three or four years old) with convulsions may be ready for the experience of nursery school. The child would be out of the home. He would be encouraged to leave his mother for a short period of time at an early age and in a natural way. He would make his first extended contact with other children. He could begin to develop the self-reliance he needs in learning to get along with others and in acquiring some self care skills such as taking off his coat and hanging it up. The play materials such as clay and finger paints are usually more varied than those available at home, and very valuable concepts in perception are formed. The children learn to differentiate textures, sizes, and colors.

Some nursery schools insist that a child be toilet-trained before attending. This rule unfortunately prevents some immature children from getting a valuable nursery school experience. This may be a difficult problem to solve for a child who is mentally retarded. Although these children are usually trained by the time they are eligible for special classes at about age seven, much valuable time has been wasted. Fortunately, many nursery schools for retarded children are being organized. Nursery schools vary from those which offer little more than group baby-sitting services to those which are imaginative and creative. It is important to be sure the child will be stimulated but not overwhelmed by the activities offered.

132 What about kindergarten?

Although many communities do not offer kindergarten in the regular public school curriculum, kindergarten attendance has many advantages. Classroom groups are usually still small, and the child who feels different because of his spells may learn to fit in with a group before he also has to tackle the problem of formal learning. He will acquire more self-help skills, he will learn to sit still for longer periods of time, and he will learn something about discipline. He will also get some preparation for reading and some number concepts. There is an increasing tendency to put more and more of the work which was taught in first grade into kindergarten; if this is the case, the parents should be very sure their child can meet the academic demands of that particular school.

There is an additional medical reason for attending kindergarten. It has to do with immunization, not education. Unless the child is the last of a large family, kindergarten will be his first exposure to a vast assortment of communicable diseases ranging from the common cold to chicken pox. He may miss a lot of school in kindergarten, but he will be building up an immunity which will come in very handy in first grade when he can really fall behind if too much work is missed. Children who take anticonvulsant medication may have difficulty maintaining an adequate daily dosage in the midst of an epidemic of vomiting and diarrhea so common among children of school age. Consultation with the child's doctor can straighten out the inevitable specific problems of medication. A mother who keeps her child at home at the slightest sign of ill-health because "he will get sick and can't take his medicine" is really handicapping his education. It is far better to learn how to cope with the problems of the routine childhood illnesses, which are bound to occur. The sooner this is done the better, and kindergarten is an excellent place to start.

**133
The
Montessori
method** The Montessori method which was developed in Italy by Maria Montessori represented a radical departure from accepted teaching methods when it was introduced about fifty years ago. The method involves letting each child learn at his own pace by mastering one standardized activity after another, according to his interests, with help and advice from the teacher. The method was used initially in teaching retarded children, but it soon was demonstrated to be successful for many children of normal intelligence. There has been a recent

revival of interest in the method. This trend seems to be a reaction against the rigid curriculum currently present in the American school system which discriminates against both the slow and the bright student.

A child who has seizures and who feels unsure of his abilities might do very well in a Montessori class. He would learn success in very small doses in an emotionally appropriate climate. A child who is a "Red Chief" with a short attention span and who has difficulty settling down would probably do better in a more structured classroom setting. This type of child usually does best under a program which follows a daily routine. To be sure, he needs a certain amount of flexibility within the routine, but he also needs to know what is going to happen next.

We are talking now about the child of normal ability whose seizures are under reasonably good control and who is about to enter first grade.

134
Can I tell if my child will be successful in a regular school?

A major question to be answered is, "Is he ready?" Different school districts have different cut-off dates for admission, but the answer to the question of readiness is not as simple as having a birthday before a particular date. Children mature at different rates academically, emotionally, and socially. Boys usually mature more slowly than girls. A child with seizures is likely to be less mature in all areas than other children his age because of his family's reactions to his problem in his home environment. The parents should ask themselves the following questions:

Is he emotionally mature? Can he meet reasonable demands without tantrums, withdrawal, or tears?

Does he understand and use words as you would expect of someone his age?

Can he feed himself, dress himself and take care of his own toilet needs?

Does he cooperate reasonably well within a group? Will he separate readily from his family and go to school eagerly?

If the answers to the questions above are affirmative, the child is right for school. But is the school right for him? Sometimes, to be sure, there is no choice about what school the child

135
The ideal school

will attend. If we consider what the *school* should be like it might make it easier to decide whether a child's lack of success is in himself or in the school.

How big are the classes? A teacher responsible for over twenty children (and this is the case in many schools) may spend a significant portion of her time just maintaining discipline. She has her hands full just trying to teach what the school district says she is supposed to teach. She has very little time to spend with the child who is learning a little more slowly than the rest of his class or with the bright child who is bored and restless. She may be especially sensitive to the actions of a child who is known to have seizures since she is afraid that the occurrence of a seizure during school would disrupt the class even more. This attitude will be sensed quickly by the child. In some very large classes a child needs only to sit still in the back of the room and behave in order to be promoted. A quiet, passive child with seizures might withdraw to avoid drawing attention to himself.

Is the curriculum flexible enough to allow for weaknesses in some areas? Most children are better in some subjects than in others. Occasionally, a bright child who is excellent in arithmetic and science is put in a slow section because his verbal skills are a little below average. The family of a child with seizures might interpret this type of placement as a direct result of his seizures, and the child himself might feel that he is being penalized because he has seizures.

Is the administration of the school enlightened about children with convulsive disorders? The attitude of the principal can do much to give the parents confidence in the school and the teachers confidence in the child. Are the teachers informed about seizures in general? Are they willing to talk over the child's problems with the parents? What is the school's policy about medication?

In some school districts, the school nurse—if there is one —is not permitted even to give aspirin. If the child needs medication in the middle of the day how will he get it? The obvious answer is either to rely on the child to take it himself or to get the doctor to change the type and timing of the medication. The parent should not, of course, use this minor obstacle as an excuse to keep the child at home.

One approach would be to tell them nothing and pretend the seizures do not exist. The reason behind this approach is "if they don't know he has convulsions they can't label him as being different." This may be true, but it is unfair to the child. Convulsions are a part of his life. They can't just be wished away. It is possible that some stress in the course of the school year will precipitate a seizure in the classroom. The confusion and anxiety this would create if no adult in the school had information about his condition would be extremely upsetting to everyone. To be sure, many children do have their first seizure in school. This is unfortunate but not preventable. The child who is known to have seizures deserves to be spared as much embarrassment as possible.

Another approach is to tell the school about the child's condition in great detail, showing considerable apprehension about the effect of stress, excess physical activity, harsh discipline, long hours, and signs of illness. Here, the mother is trying to make her problem the school's problem, but the *school* is not responsible for controlling the spells. This represents the other extreme and is just as wrong. The convulsions must be kept in perspective. The school should be informed in a matter-of-fact way. Sometimes it is wise to wait a few weeks if the seizures are well controlled. Then at a conference with the teacher the mother can say "I'm so pleased with the way Johnny is getting along. He used to have spells, and he still takes medicine for them. They certainly don't seem to have affected him in any way." The teacher will be forced to agree and her initial reaction to the information will be positive. Often a note which briefly summarizes the problem from the family doctor to the school is very helpful.

136
What should I tell the school about his condition?

The answer to this question is usually **NO**. Although a tranquilizer might slow him down physically for a short period of time, it may not help him to learn. Tranquilizers may decrease his movement, but acquisition of knowledge is a much more complicated process than just sitting still. Sometimes a doctor prescribes a tranquilizer as a possible quick solution to a complicated problem. He, too, needs to feel he is helping in some way, and perhaps a tranquilizer *might* work. Sometimes a teacher will suggest that a mother ask her doctor to pre-

137
My child is very restless. Could tranquilizers help him learn?

scribe one. Perhaps it will get the child to sit still; a deeper reason may be her desire to calm him down and keep him out of the way so that the rest of the children can be taught. Perhaps the mother hopes he will be quieter around the house as well.

The tranquilizer is rarely actually intended for the child. It may really be subconsciously intended for the parent, the teacher, or the doctor who prescribes it. A very few children with uncontrollable hyperactivity may benefit from one of the amphetamine compounds. Although these drugs are stimulants, they may quiet the child by making him less responsive to all the stimuli around him. Somehow his energy is channeled and he no longer overreacts to his immediate environment. There is as yet no real agreement about the actual benefits of this drug. In my opinion, the number of children in whom its use might be successful is very small.

The solution may be quite complicated. Perhaps the child is bored; perhaps he is overwhelmed and frustrated by inability to do the work; perhaps he has cerebral dysfunction [101–103] and cannot fit into a large group. Whatever the reason, the solution does not often lie in a magic pill.

138
Should he be
in a special
class?
Most school districts have special classes for "retarded educable" children. The teachers are specially trained to teach this type of child and many of them are remarkably competent, patient, and wise. An attempt is made to teach the children as many of the basic academic skills as they can master. It often turns out to be a rather surprising amount. I remember an eleven-year-old boy who spent five years in a retarded educable class. He then went into a regular grade where he was able to do all the work. He was a little older than the rest of the class, but he was able to adjust well. Not all of the children do this well, but the teachers try to get them to function to the best of their ability.

They learn to sit quietly, to pay attention and to follow directions. At first, a very small amount of correct work brings a reward such as a gold star; later the amount is gradually increased so that the child learns to work with persistence and sustained effort in pursuit of a reward. This training is invaluable when the time comes to seek a job. In many ways it is more important than being able to read at grade level. In most school districts, a child qualifies for special education if he has a certain minimal IQ, and no provision is made for those whose IQs are below that level. A recent court decision in Pennsylvania may change the situation, so that *all* children must be educated. In Philadelphia, children with IQs over 50 are eligible. There are also classes for trainable children with IQs between 25 and 50. Privately-owned schools are likely to be more flexible about admission policies.

The ideal special class will have a relatively small number of students, who are fairly compatible. The teacher will plan the work extremely carefully to meet the children's needs. These needs may vary from week to week, and she must plan ahead and yet remain flexible. In some poorly run, poorly equipped, and underfinanced school districts, special classes are nothing more than an unselected group of a great variety of children whose needs cannot possibly be met by one teacher. A 16-year-old severely retarded boy might be in the same classroom with an emotionally disturbed eight-year-old girl who had no place else to go. This type of facility is worthless, and pressure should be brought on the school administration to change it.

A child who is mentally retarded and who has seizures is unlikely to encounter any great social difficulties in a well-organized special class. The children are recognized as individuals; each one has some sort of handicap, and the emphasis on conformity found in regular classes has given way to an earnest attempt to help each individual child achieve success.

139
The day care center

In addition to facilities for working mothers, many communities have day care centers which provide a form of training for those children who are too handicapped to go into a special class. In a day care center, the emphasis is on self-care, social skills, and awareness of oneself as a person. The children learn to put on coats, sweaters, and boots. They learn their own names and the names of the other pupils in the class. They learn names of objects and the parts of the body. They enjoy rhythm and music and learn to eat without spilling. Adequate personnel is a key factor in the success of a day care center. There must be someone to help pass out the juice and cookies and help the children drink if necessary; there must be someone who can take an active, noisy child aside so that the teacher can work with the others; someone must help in the bathroom and help put on coats and sweaters. Some day care centers are part of the county or municipal school system. Some are privately owned.

A retarded child with convulsions will get a great deal out of a good day care center. He gets out of the house; he has a regular routine; he learns some basic skills which make his care easier for others. If he is busy and happy his seizures are likely to diminish in number and severity. The atmosphere of a day care center is likely to be friendly and the seizures of a retarded child will be kept in perspective as merely part of the problem.

A day care facility near Philadelphia, which also operates as a day camp in the summer, has an ingenious system for sorting out a large number of children according to age and ability without using such disagreeable terms as "low-grade," "high-grade," or "trainable." The groups are given the names of birds. The staff knows there is a pecking order, but the children are quite content to be canaries, robins, or parakeets.

**140
Living away
from home** Occasionally a severely handicapped child needs a great deal of care, and there is no facility in the area which can meet his needs on a daytime basis. The question of placement in some sort of institution which could do more for him then arises. Routine, activity, and freedom from stress could help to improve behavior to reduce the frequency of seizures. The family may feel he could get these if he were cared for elsewhere. Unfortunately there are not enough institutions. Many are crowded, antiquated, remote, or expensive; many have long waiting lists. The family must decide whether the advantage to the child justifies a possible financial sacrifice which could affect their other children, and whether the child would indeed be happier away from his family. Sometimes the family feels the child should be placed out of the home "for the sake of the other children." There are usually other reasons which are more important.

A close family may or may not be affected adversely by the presence of a severely handicapped child. In many cases, it brings them closer together and encourages responsibility and compassion in the other children at an early age. A severely handicapped child could, on the other hand, be really disturbing in a family already beset by major tensions and problems. The child's size may make him unmanageable. The limitation of space at home and lack of facilities in the community may force institutional care. Temporary placement out of the home may be a better solution if the right place can be found.

An Amish farmer once discussed the problem of his severely retarded nine-year-old son with me. The local health authorities had felt that the boy might benefit from systematic training at a day care center ten miles away. The father would have no part of it. His reasoning was extremely sound. The boy was one of ten children. His convulsions had not been a problem for several years. He was very much a cherished member of the family. He was kept occupied by watching and sometimes helping with the farm chores. There was always someone available to make sure he did not hurt himself or wander off. The family had taught him to dress himself, to feed himself and to care for his toilet needs. His days were happy and full. "You can teach anybody anything if you just have patience," his father concluded. He was so right, and I agreed with him completely. In a different family, in different surroundings, this boy might have needed at least a day care center. Some families with less skill and patience would have considered putting him in an institution. The actual mental ability and the severity of the convulsions are not the only deciding factors in determining where a child should be. The attitude and personality of the family and the community environment are also important. Sometimes professional help may be needed to assist the family in making this difficult decision.

141
Is education out of the home always necessary?

FUTURE PLANNING

Proper upbringing of any child involves the development of reliability, independence, and the ability to get along well with others. These qualities are necessary if a child is to lead a

142

successful and productive life—they are also vitally important in determining successful vocational placement. Vocational guidance starts, therefore, before the child goes to school for the first time. Schooling will develop specific skills, but reliability, independence, and the ability to get along well with others must be encouraged at home.

These qualities must be sought within the limits of the individual's abilities, but these abilities must be allowed to develop. Children with seizures are likely to be protected from experiences which will allow them to solve problems without interference. They tend to ask for help from an adult who is likely to be nearby in case the child has a seizure. They tend to prefer the company of adults rather than peers. Athletic competition may be only partially successful as a way they can learn to obey rules and participate in group activities. The child with seizures may be accepted by his peers not for himself but because they feel sorry for him. After years of this kind of unfortunate conditioning, the child with seizures may suddenly be asked to select a vocation just because he has reached a certain age. Any vocational placement will be uncertain and unrealistic unless positive efforts toward character building have been made all along [121, 122].

A young adult's skills and character should be evaluated several years before he reaches the age at which the school system ends its responsibilities. The guidance counselor will evaluate a youngster's reliability, social behavior, ability to take criticism, and problem-solving abilities. He will evaluate his special skills. The questions of possible limitations because of his chronic seizures will then be examined. How well controlled are his seizures? What kind of transportation can he use? It is wise for the individual to gain experience in a limited way before he is suddenly turned loose in the world.

The type of work the child eventually does and the type of life he will lead depends of course on his own skills and the extent of his handicap. He should be able to work at something at which he is competent, which brings him satisfaction, and which benefits the community in some way. It is hoped that the job will enable him to be partly or wholly self-supporting. A young adult with convulsions must consider another factor. He cannot work in any position where he will put himself in danger or possibly endanger the lives of others. Certain types of factory work with open machinery would be dangerous. Window washing and house painting would be unwise choices. A person with convulsions cannot be licensed as a commercial pilot, but is not prevented from holding a private pilot's license. He cannot serve in the armed forces according to present regulations.

Just as a child with seizures must be successful in a classroom situation, a young adult must be successful in his job. The job must be right for him. He, too, is singled out because of his seizures, and he too is sensitive to surrounding attitudes. Intelligence is merely one of several attributes which must be considered in proper job placement. Personality is very important. How well does he get along with people? If he tends to be a loner he had better not be in a position where he meets the public. Is he punctual? Is he dependable? How much supervision does he need? Someone might be perfectly capable of maintaining a corner newsstand but he would not be able to take the responsibility of stocking it and making it a profitable business. He would be better off doing factory work where there are no real decisions to be made. A person who has seizures might lose out to a person of similar ability without seizures simply because he cannot cope with getting to the job by car or by public transportation although he might do the job better than the other applicant.

Many young men and women are overwhelmed by a high-pressure, fast-moving urban or suburban environment. No job seems right, and they are discouraged by the negative attitude they meet. These individuals could get along very well in a quieter, noncompetitive rural area where they would not be singled out and where they could manage most of the work with a gain in self-respect brought about by the respect of others. Sometimes a young adult is guided to an appropriate opportunity (for example, a sheltered workshop), but the adults who know him and are still responsible for his care undermine his successful adjustment. They may feel he is associating with undesirable people; they may resent the social stigma often associated with sheltered workshops; they may scoff at the low pay and they may say that he is too bright for that kind of job. Guidance from home as well as from professionals is necessary.

Vocational planning must be realistic. The vocation for which he is being trained should be one for which there is a real demand and which is in little immediate danger of becoming obsolete because of automation.

Even though great medical progress has been made in the treatment of recurrent seizures, the attitudes of employers toward a known epileptic may still be very negative. There is no evidence that workers with well-controlled seizures are any more accident prone than anyone else, but the employer may be afraid his Workmen's Compensation costs will rise. Much needs to be done to educate employers that a person with a controlled seizure disorder is a dependable worker *if the job is otherwise appropriate for him.*

143
College

If a youngster has the intellectual ability to go to college and if he is considered emotionally and socially mature enough, the presence of seizures is no detriment. College students are under various types of stress. A boy whose seizures were under excellent control at home with a routine of regular hours, good food, and some parental supervision of activities may have a temporary increase in the number of spells at college. He stays up 'til all hours; his meals are irregular, he worries about his work, and he must make decisions. Control of his spells may be difficult until he gets used to this new way of life.

Exam time is a particularly stressful period. College physicians have learned to expect a few students to have their first convulsion during mid-year exams of their freshman year. The condition, long latent, is apparently triggered by the stress surrounding exams.

144
Filling out
application
forms

Many routine forms have questions concerning the applicant's past medical history. These may include fainting, fits, convulsions, or epilepsy. If the persons who have access to this information were always intelligent and enlightened, the questions would be easy to answer. This cannot be assumed, and considerable discretion is needed. It should also be recognized that the policy of a large company against hiring an

individual with seizures cannot be altered by a local repre-
sentative.

Obviously, no individual should apply for a position that
would be hazardous for him or for others. If the applicant is
well placed, the fact that he receives medication will rarely
cause his discharge even if it becomes known at some future
time. It may even be an advantage to the employer who will
recognize the fact that the person whose seizures are well
controlled will be less likely to seek employment elsewhere.
The underlying problem is that the employer (or his agent)
is at first reluctant to take a chance. His worries are generally
vague and nonspecific. They are therefore difficult to answer.
He may be worried about his insurance, his responsibilities,
and what would happen if a seizure did occur. On the other
hand an employer might hire the same individual if the space
on the form is checked off as "none." After an individual has
been turned down because he has answered the question
precisely, there is very little he can do.

If the question "Have you ever lost consciousness?"
were answered honestly by everyone, one reply in ten would
be "Yes." What is really intended by the question is "Do you
have recurrent episodes of unconsciousness that are likely
to interfere in the performance of this job?" If the answer is
yes, then by all means the situation should be discussed and
possibly a trial worked out on a mutually acceptable basis. If
the answer is no, then the employer does not need to be
involved. He does not expect or want to be; he has enough
worries of his own without those of someone else.

For college applications the same concepts are needed.
If the individual is likely to have difficulty in college because
recurrent episodes of unconsciousness are likely to occur,
then the special situation must be worked out. If the physician
in the student health department will have some kind of
responsibility (such as renewing prescriptions or obtaining
blood counts), the individual's physician at home will want to
make these arrangements directly. This information need
not be in the registrar's office. It is medical information and
is not a part of a student's academic record. Physicians of
student health departments respect the confidential nature of
various problems which come to their attention. After ad-

mission to the college, the health needs of the students are solved on an individual basis.

145
Marriage
In a way, marriage is just as important a part of the work of life as is a suitable job or career. In fact, in our society marriage for a girl may be the job for which she has been educated. The presence of reasonably well-controlled convulsions has little to do with the success of a marriage, provided the individual is ready for marriage in other ways. Is her health good? Is she emotionally stable? Does she have the mental capacity to keep the house properly? In the case of a young man one must also ask if he is self-supporting, and if his prospects for continued employment are good? These factors are important. The seizures are not. Until fairly recently, the prevailing attitude toward seizures was one of ignorance and fear. Until recently there were actually laws forbidding an epileptic to marry in some states. Fortunately, they have all been repealed.

146
Are seizures hereditary?
Most seizures are not hereditary, however there are some particular types of seizures which are inherited, particularly those of the petit mal variety [67]. There is no real agreement about whether other types are hereditary. Some families appear to have a predisposition toward seizures, but the causes of seizures are so varied and so numerous it is impossible to be certain.

As long as the prospective parents are healthy, emotionally stable, and have the mental ability and financial resources to bring up a child, there is no reason why the presence of controlled convulsions should be an obstacle to parenthood. Women with a history of convulsions do perfectly well during childbirth and can even breast feed their infants if they so desire. The anticonvulsant medication will not affect the baby. It is a well-known medical fact that children with convulsions remain under better control and get along better in their environment if one or both parents happen to have had seizures. Probably these parents are able to draw on their own experiences in a constructive way.

147
Community environment
The environment which will affect a child with seizures consists of the home, the school, and the community. The community can provide physical resources which may benefit a

child with seizures, and it will also provide an attitude which will affect him. The two are really interdependent. The attitude in the community will determine what kind of facilities (including schools, parks, and recreational areas) are available. The quality of these resources will inevitably affect the academic and social progress in that community of the child with seizures.

The ideal community will have adequate resources for all mental health needs. I can list those most needed for a child with seizures:

**148
What
resources
should be
present?**

A diagnostic center.   There should be a medical facility where specialists can be consulted for help. A child with seizures might need rather complicated laboratory studies, x-rays, EEGs, and psychological evaluations. An evaluation at this diagnostic center should be within the means of all who seek help. The center should maintain cordial relations with the physicians in the community, and free communication should be encouraged.

The school system.   The school system should provide the type of education in regular classes which can be well utilized by the child with seizures [135]. There should be remedial help available, and there should be classes for children with cerebral dysfunction or specific learning disabilities. Special education classes within the school system should be of two types. One type will train mildly retarded pupils, some of whom have seizures, to become self-sufficient adult citizens. The other will train moderately retarded pupils, who also may have seizures, to become partially self-sufficient in protected settings.

Day care or regional centers. [See also 139]   A day care center should be set up for those who cannot profit from formal training. In Connecticut, for example, facilities for 24-hour care have been helpful. Most children with seizures or other handicapping conditions can best be cared for at home, in foster homes, or in centers with ample facilities. However, the problems of transportation, inadequate budgets, and the like are often formidable.

Vocational counseling.   Vocational counseling, job training, and placement services should be available since a young
adult with seizures may have considerable difficulty in finding
just the right job [142].

Public health nurse and homemaker services.   Sometimes
a child with seizures is severely physically and mentally handicapped. Accident or illness in the family might make the
child's care an intolerable burden. A public health nurse can
be of specific help in the physical care of the child or of the
injured or ill member of the family when such a situation
arises. Many public health nurses provide invaluable moral
support as well.

Counseling.   Many families find that they need outside
professional help in sorting out their feelings toward the
convulsions and toward the child who has them. There may
be difficult decisions about schooling or placement outside the
home. There may be feelings of guilt or hostility toward the
child. Sometimes counseling is available at a diagnostic center;
sometimes it may be obtained from another community
agency [148, 149].

Residential centers.   Some children with seizures present
problems of care and training so complex that the home
environment will no longer suffice [140]. Temporary placement in a residential center may be the answer if the family
can be taught to improve the situation at home so that the
youngster can fit in on return. Sometimes permanent placement in a residential center is the only solution.

The residential center should be modern, efficient, and of
sufficient size to meet the community needs but small enough
to ensure adequate personnel. The outlook should be positive
with an emphasis on rehabilitation and training rather than
on simple custodial care. Often a planned separation of five
days a week or one month each year has real advantages for
both the child and his family.

Plans for new residential centers should include placing
multiple small facilities throughout the state, each serving a
group of communities. The family is then never too far away

from the child, and the child is never too far from the community into which he may hope to return. The traditional state hospital, a big barn-like structure housing 1500 or more people, is inefficient, expensive, and obsolete.

In some hospitals, medical social workers are responsible for financial arrangements and for transfer of patients to convalescent facilities. Professional workers who have degrees in social work and who have earned ACSW (Academy Certified Social Workers) certificates usually have broader responsibilities. They know how to use the facilities of the community and understand the impact of a problem on the family unit. A social worker either in a medical setting or in an agency for families or children is often in a good position to help work out realistic solutions for many difficult situations. In our pediatric clinic, consultation with a social worker is usually initiated by a physician. He suggests that the social worker and the parent agree to discuss a particular problem. Sometimes parents can be helped by being in a group with other parents who have children with similar difficulties. The social worker does not start with a preconceived notion but helps the family work out the solution which is best for them.

For example, a mother who has entered her child in nursery school may be concerned that the child will cry when she leaves him. This may be easily resolved during one interview. Sometimes the anxiety associated with separation requires considerable effort by both the parent and the worker because other problems may need to be solved first. One of these may be the fact that the child has had seizures in the past.

Sometimes a social service worker can be instrumental in helping parents discuss the implications of seizures with their children. In other instances the need is for the parents to see their child in perspective and not to allow the seizure disorder to become the major focus of all parental concern. The positive aspects of the child's development need to be discovered and emphasized. The physician's reassurance may not be enough. The social service worker helps parents understand the basis for the child's actions and the parents' feelings toward them.

149
What is the role of the social worker?

Allan, age 13, became restless in school and at home; it was impossible for anyone to discipline him effectively; he became unable to concentrate on his school work. It was found that he thought that his spells meant that he was crazy. Unfortunately, every effort on his part to talk to his father about the spells was met with evasion on the part of his father and reassurance on the part of his mother. After the parents were helped to see that Allan was being left to struggle alone with the problem, they were able to find ways of meeting his needs realistically. In this instance his school and disciplinary problems could not be handled effectively until his parents learned to work together.

Billy, age 12, was a frequent school truant. When his mother found out and confronted him, she discovered that he was afraid of what the reaction of the other children might be if he had a spell in school. He had been afraid to talk to her about it because she had never shown any readiness to discuss his seizures with him. The social worker helped her clarify her own feelings about the seizures so that she could discuss them more freely with her son.

150
Realities

Unfortunately the services outlined above exist in very few communities. The failure of most communities to meet these needs is caused by a tangled mess of politics, inept administrative policies, inadequate finances, ignorance, and apathy. These community services are provided by different levels of government. Traditionally, the state runs the residential centers; the local communities run the schools. The overall planning may be in the hands of a state department of mental health or a department of welfare. There is an inevitable squabble over how much state money is allocated for services in a large city. Public health services may be run at a state level, a county level, or a city level—in some cases, all three governments are involved. There is never enough money. What money there is is often not spent wisely. Sometimes there is a duplication of services; sometimes there is no facility where a child can get a particular service.

State or local governments may be behind the times. For example, millions of dollars might be earmarked to update and renovate a state hospital which is nothing more than a seventy-five year old overcrowded warehouse of 1500 people. The money should have been spent five years earlier to build multiple small residential centers and half-way houses thereby phasing out the obsolete facility before it became uninhabitable.

Some of the smaller states such as Connecticut have done relatively well in planning and financing their resources. One state (Massachusetts) will provide out-of-state tuition for a child who has an emotional disturbance with or without convulsions if the facility is accredited and if a place is not available within the state.

A well-organized group may lobby effectively at the state level in a larger state for one particular type of facility. Funds which would do more good spread out in diverse activities may therefore be funneled into one particular aspect of mental health, to the detriment of others.

Voluntary profit-making and nonprofit organizations can meet some of these community needs. These facilities may also have problems of restrictive or misguided administration. One mildly retarded five-year-old boy with fairly well-controlled seizures was turned down by a particular nursery school because he did not have a "physical handicap." This particular nursery school "for physically handicapped" children of all mental levels was supported by community funds. Yet this member of the community was refused because he did not have a *limp*. An excellent church-supported residential center which provides loving care to severely physically and mentally handicapped children refuses children with seizures. The private facilities which provide the best service have usually been organized in response to a definite community need and do not offer their services to any but those who fit into the specific category which they were created to serve.

There is no easy way to bridge the gap between optimal community resources and what is really found. The most helpful solutions lie in the persistent determined efforts of groups of parents of children with seizures or any other chronic problems to work for change. These efforts can take the form of organizing the community to provide the service by nudging the local, state, or federal government to fill the need. Constant dissemination of information about the problems and their immediate needs is required at the local or governmental level. The spread of this information and the dialogue initiated between the concerned parents and the community will, in themselves, be a partial solution. Out of shared information and communication can come an awareness of the problems and an atmosphere which challenges traditional beliefs. These changes of attitude in the community will ultimately benefit the child.

APPENDIX 1
CLASSIFICATION OF
CONVULSIVE DISORDERS
BY CAUSE

I. Acute or nonrecurrent forms
   A. Febrile convulsions (eg, at the beginning of infections out-
      side the nervous system or in association with high environ-
      mental temperatures).
   B. Infections within the central nervous system (eg, meningitis,
      encephalitis, brain abscess, tetanus, malaria, typhus fever).
   C. Brain hemorrhage
      (eg, from birth injury, bleeding disorders such as hemophilia,
      rupture of blood vessels, sickle cell disease).
   D. Poisoning
      1. Drugs which can cause convulsions such as strychnine,
         camphor, certain antihistamines, certain tranquilizers.
      2. Bacterial poisons (eg, certain forms of dysentery).
      3. Lead, arsenic.
   E. Sudden oxygen deprivation (eg, near-drowning, inhalation
      anesthesia).
   F. Metabolic disturbances in body chemistry (eg, tetany, hypo-
      glycemia, certain vitamin deficiencies).
   G. Sudden swelling of the brain from water retention (eg, kid-
      ney disease).
   H. Brain tumor.
   I. Miscellaneous diseases (eg, porphyria).

Adapted from: Baird, H. W., In: *Textbook of Pediatrics*, 9th Edition, Ed.
by W. E. Nelson, V. C. Vaughan, R. McKay. Philadelphia, W. B. Saun-
ders, 1969.

II. Chronic or recurrent forms
  A. Epilepsy
    1. Idiopathic (also called primary, cryptogenic, essential or genuine epilepsy).
    2. Organic (also called secondary or symptomatic epilepsy) with residual brain damage from previous injuries, insults, or infections.
      a. Organic epilepsy may follow:
        1) direct laceration of brain tissue; 2) bleeding within the brain from birth injury, accident, rupture of blood vessel; 3) severe sudden deprivation of oxygen; and 4) infections: encephalitis, meningitis, abscess, hypoglycemia, poisoning by lead or arsenic.
      b. Organic epilepsy may be caused by:
        1) degenerative diseases of the central nervous system; 2) congenital malformations of the brain; 3) parasitic brain diseases (eg, syphilis); and 4) sensations: touch, light, sound, self-induced.
  B. Epilepsy-simulating states:
    1. Narcolepsy
    2. Hysteria
    3. Tetany (low calcium)
    4. Hypoglycemic states
    5. Uremia
    6. Syncopal attacks (eg, simple fainting attacks, hyperactive carotid sinus reflex)
    7. Migraine and abdominal epilepsy.

APPENDIX 2

WHAT IS KNOWN ABOUT THE ORIGIN OF BRAIN WAVES AND THE CHEMICAL MECHANISM FOR SEIZURES?

The results of investigations in invertebrate animals suggest that brain waves have the same rhythm as movement of the gills in primitive species, like the shark. This and other evidence indicates that as additional parts of the central nervous system evolved, different rhythms developed. It seems likely that very little of the preexisting nervous system was discarded and that the new rhythms became superimposed upon those already present, rather than replacing them. The specializations of the newly formed portions of the central nervous system also seem to involve more complex ways of storing and releasing energy.

Clinical seizures arise because the stability of a cell membrane (or wall) is damaged. The leak or break results in excessive or prolonged release of energy (excessive depolarization). In man, the repair to the leak (repolarization) probably depends upon a chemical reaction involving "high energy" phosphate compounds which are naturally present in the cells and respond quickly in order to preserve the balance of potassium and sodium across the cell wall. If excessive bombardment of energy from a damaged or leaking cell continues, neighboring cells become involved, and alterations in many cells and their connections take place. Anticonvulsant medications probably act by stabilizing the cell membrane so that excessive, repetitive discharges are less likely to occur.

APPENDIX 3
EPILEPSY AND DRIVING

GUIDE ISSUED BY THE AMERICAN MEDICAL
ASSOCIATION COMMITTEE ON MEDICAL ASPECTS
OF AUTOMOTIVE SAFETY (1968) [1]

Neurological Disorders. Convulsive disorders, including grave or petit seizures, or psychomotor epilepsy are the most frequently encountered neurological disorders which can impair driving ability.

Epileptic patients who have been seizure-free for at least a year, and who are reliable in taking their medications, are considered good risks for the operation of private vehicles, but should be advised not to drive commercial or passenger transport vehicles. Physicians should inform patients regarding the potential hazards of the drugs they are taking.

Epileptic patients should not consume alcoholic beverages in any form for at least 24 hours prior to driving. Fatigue should be avoided, and six hours should be the maximum behind the wheel in one day. Also, those who are subject to photic stimuli should be advised that night driving carries added danger because opposing headlights may precipitate a seizure. Emotional stress should be minimized by avoiding driving in peak traffic hours.

Epileptic patients should have frequent medical review of their condition, and even those who have been seizure-free for more than a year should be evaluated every six months.

---

[1] From "Physician's Guide for Determining Driver Limitation," Chicago: American Medical Association, 1968, p. 15. Reprinted with the permission of the American Medical Association.

APPENDIX 4
SUMMARY OF
DRIVER'S LICENSE LAWS

All states grant licenses to epileptics who supply satisfactory evidence that their seizures have been under control for a reasonable time and that they can operate a motor vehicle with reasonable safety. The details of what evidence is needed to satisfy the state statutes vary widely from state to state.

The statutes of most states prohibit licensing of persons who for a variety of reasons would be unsafe drivers. Administrators of driver's licensing laws may, in addition, impose certain qualifications for applicants with epilepsy. Others have specific statutory regulations concerning issuance of licenses to drivers with epilepsy.

Epileptics covered only under general "unsafe driver" category; discretionary regulation (12): Arkansas, Washington, D. C., Maryland, Mississippi, Missouri, Nebraska, New Mexico, Oklahoma, Rhode Island, Texas, Vermont, Wyoming.

Epileptics licensed on physician's recommendation or "judicial decree" (22): Alabama, Alaska, Arizona, California, Delaware, Georgia, Hawaii, Idaho, Illinois, Iowa, Louisiana, North Carolina, North Dakota, Ohio (6 mo license), Oregon, South Carolina, South Dakota, Tennessee, Texas, Utah, Virginia, Wisconsin (6 mo license).

One-year seizure-free period required (8): Colorado, Indiana, Kansas, Kentucky, Maine, Michigan, Nevada, Washington.

Eighteen-month seizure-free period required (2): Massachusetts, New Hampshire.

Two-year seizure-free period required (8): Connecticut, Florida,

(Adapted from "The Legal Rights of Persons with Epilepsy." Published by the Epilepsy Foundation, 1965.)

Minnesota, Montana, New Jersey, New York (3 years for permanent license), Pennsylvania, West Virginia.

Alabama: Licensing of any person . . . suffering from a physical or mental disability which . . . will prevent such persons from exercising reasonable control over a motor vehicle is prohibited. Administration requires that epileptics furnish administrator annual certificates from family physician.

Alaska: Administrator licenses epileptic only on receipt of physician's recommendation and imposes restriction "Medical certification required for renewal."

Arizona: Licensing of applicants whose driving would be harmful to public safety is prohibited. Administrator has authority to give a physical and mental examination "to determine the applicant's fitness to safely operate . . . a motor vehicle." He *may* place restrictions upon the applicant with respect to where and when he will drive. Physician's letter is a requirement for application.

Arkansas: Administrator may give such examinations as are found necessary "to determine the applicant's fitness to operate . . . a motor vehicle safely." Restrictions may be imposed.

California: Applicants may be licensed "if a physical or mental defect does not affect driving ability." Licenses may be issued for limited terms and/or with restrictions. Reinstatement of revoked licenses possible on probationary basis with periodic reports from physician.

Colorado: An epileptic applicant must present a certificate noting that he has been seizure-free for one year. A Medical Advisory Committee advises on questionable applications.

Connecticut: Applicants must be seizure-free for at least two years. Thereafter, a medical statement must be filed periodically to show that the operator has remained seizure-free. Limited licenses may be issued. No appeal possible from decision of the administrator.

Delaware: "Declared epileptics who have not been restored to competency by judicial decree or released from the hospital with the superintendent's certification . . . are denied licenses." Only uncontrollable cases are reported to the Motor Vehicle Department. Delaware State Hospital makes decisions as to whether a person will continue to be licensed.

District of Columbia: No specific laws regarding epilepsy. Administrator may withhold a license where public safety is endangered.

Florida: Applicants must be seizure-free for two years before they are issued licenses. Once issued a license, they must submit reports for license renewal for two years before this requirement is lifted.

Georgia: Issuance of licenses to persons unable to safely operate a motor vehicle prohibited. Any individual subject to seizures must furnish a complete medical history to the Department of Public Safety.

Hawaii: Administrator is required "to make such examination as necessary to determine the applicant's physical and mental abilities to operate a motor vehicle safely." Driver's licenses are *not* issued to people who are subject to epileptic seizures. Suspension of license pending a physician's certificate.

Idaho: "Controlling medication at all times" is the restriction placed on some epileptic licensees, and the licenses are renewed each six months if licensee remains seizure-free.

Illinois: "The Secretary of State shall not issue or renew any license . . . to any person who is or has been afflicted with epilepsy unless such person shall furnish to the Secretary of State a verified written statement . . . from a competent medical specialist . . ." stating that the applicant can safely operate a motor vehicle.

Certification of control with or without medication is adequate if there is no longer any doubt that the applicant may suffer an attack when driving.

Indiana: "Adjudged epileptics cannot be licensed until restored to competency by judicial decree or release from the hospital with certificate of competency." Medical statement from a physician showing that the person has been free of lapses of consciousness for one year is required.

Iowa: "Persons who would not be safe drivers by reason of physical or mental disabilities are prohibited from licensing." Where such disabilities exist, an examination may be required. Operator's privileges only given after assurance that the person will not suffer attacks while driving.

Kansas: If the applicant states on his application that he is afflicted with a physical or mental disability, he must pass an examination before being licensed.

If an epileptic becomes involved in an accident, his license is cancelled and reinstated only after a statement from the physician that he has been seizure-free for at least one year.

Kentucky: "Adjudged epileptics cannot be issued licenses until they are restored to competency by judicial decree or released from a hospital with a certificate of competency." With a past history of epilepsy, applicants must provide a physician's certification of control of seizures. Freedom from seizures for one year is considered sufficient for issuance of a license.

Louisiana: Administrator may withhold or revoke licenses where individual is deemed unable to drive safely by reason of physical or mental disability. Medical statement as to the frequency and severity of seizures and whether they are controllable is required.

Maine: All applicants must pass a physical examination. Epileptics are required to present certification from physician that they are controlled or seizure-free for one year or more. "When such certification is made, a license is issued with the restriction that the applicant maintain the use of the medication prescribed."

Maryland: A Medical Advisory Board reviews each case with a medical problem individually, without preexisting rules and regulations.

Massachusetts: "Persons with 'epileptic-form type of seizures' are issued licenses upon report of a neurologist that the applicant has been seizure-free for at least 18 months." Applicant must furnish periodic reports from the same neurologist.

Michigan: "Licenses cannot be issued to applicants who have previously been adjudged epileptics and who have not . . . been restored to competency by judicial decree." Licenses are issued when an applicant has been controlled for at least one year without any attacks. Immediate review is given where a person is reported to have been involved in an accident or lost consciousness.

Minnesota: "Prohibition of licensing a person previously adjudged epileptic unless the administrator is satisfied that the person is competent in operating a motor vehicle." Statement from physician required stating that applicant has been free from seizures for at least two years, and that attacks in the future are unlikely.

Mississippi: Licensing at the discretion of the director of the Department of Motor Vehicles. A.M.A. Guidelines are followed.

Missouri: If the applicant's fitness to operate a motor vehicle safely is questioned, physical and mental examination by a licensed physician may be required.

Montana: "The Board may issue a license to a person suffering from epileptic seizures when the afflicted person can show he has been seizure-free . . . for two years."

Nebraska: No statutory provisions specifically pertaining to epileptics. All applicants with a physical defect must pass a physical examination.

Nevada: "The administrator requires certification from treating physician that an epileptic applicant has had his condition cured or arrested by medication and has been seizure-free for at least one year."

New Hampshire: The Motor Vehicle Department does not issue a license until the person has been controlled by medication for 18 months with confirmed information from the Board of Health.

New Jersey: "A person who has . . . suffered from seizures . . . may be licensed when he has been seizure-free for two years with or without medication." An EEG and a statement from his physician and the Advisory Council for Convulsive Disorders must accompany the application. Reports must also be submitted at six-month intervals.

New Mexico: "Epileptics may be licensed at the discretion of the Commissioner. If doubt exists, the Commissioner or applicant may request a review of the case by a medical advisory committee."

New York: Applicants must be free from seizures for two years, with or without medication. Statements from both the family physician and a specialist are required, as well as periodic medical reports. The applicant must agree to refrain from the use of alcoholic beverages. Persons free from seizures for three years may be granted a license without further periodic medical reports.

North Carolina: "A license will not be issued to a grand mal epileptic unless he has been restored to competency by judicial decree or has a certification. A license is also refused "where physical disability prevents the applicant from exercising reasonable control over a vehicle."

North Dakota: A license is granted to persons with histories of epilepsy whose physicians certify that the condition is controlled.

Oklahoma: A license is refused "to any person afflicted with . . . a physical condition that would impair the driving ability of such a person."

Ohio: Six-month licenses are issued for persons whose epileptic condition is either dormant or under medical control.

Oregon: "A license cannot be issued to anyone who is afflicted with or subject to any condition which brings about momentary or prolonged lapses of consciousness or control, which is or may become chronic, or when such person is . . . unable to exercise reasonable control over a motor vehicle."

Pennsylvania: "Adjudged epileptics cannot be licensed until restored to competency by judicial decree or certified by a hospital. Two years freedom from an attack with or without medication is required of a person with a history of epilepsy."

Rhode Island: No specific regulations regarding epileptics. Anyone who, because of physical or mental disability, is unable to safely operate a motor vehicle is denied a license.

South Carolina: No licensing of persons who are not safe drivers because of mental or physical disabilities. Epileptics must furnish semiannual medical statements. Examinations may be given to determine capabilities.

South Dakota: "The Commission cannot issue a license to anyone who will not be a safe driver. Medical certification of an epileptic's ability to drive is required, and a restricted license stating *Epileptic; epilepsy controlled by medication* is issued."

Tennessee: No licenses are issued to anyone the Commissioner feels would be an unsafe driver. Epileptics are issued licenses "if it is medically established that their condition is under control."

Texas: A license may be issued to epileptics if a physician verifies that the condition is under control and that the applicant would be a safe driver.

Utah: Those applicants who have ever suffered from epilepsy must furnish a physician's statement indicating whether they are physically qualified to drive before a license may be issued.

Vermont: No specific statutes regarding epilepsy. Commissioner refuses licenses to those he feels to be physically unfit to be safe drivers. A medical examination may be ordered, and a restricted license may be issued.

Virginia: "Adjudged epileptics cannot be licensed until restored to competency by judicial decree or released from a mental institution with a certificate of competency." Generally, epileptics must provide periodic statements of their physical conditions from their physicians.

Washington: "Adjudged epileptics cannot be licensed until restored to competency by judicial decree or released from a hospital with a certificate of competency." Restricted license may be issued. The applicant must submit a medical statement showing that he has been seizure-free for one year and that his condition is controlled by medication. Periodic check-ups required.

West Virginia: Before licensing, anyone with a physical disability must present a letter from his physician as to the severity of his illness. An epileptic must be seizure-free for two years and be controlled by medication.

Wisconsin: Only temporary licenses issued to epileptics. They are effective for 6 months, renewable upon presentation of a physician's statement stating that the applicant is on medication and has been seizure-free and able to safely operate a motor vehicle.

Wyoming: No specific regulations regarding epileptics.

APPENDIX 5
GLOSSARY

abdominal epilepsy: a form of childhood migraine accompanied by nausea, vomiting, and severe abdominal pain.

adrenocorticotropic hormone: an organic substance, secreted by the pituitary gland, which stimulates the outer portion of the adrenal gland; it is sometimes used in the treatment of infantile myoclonic seizures.

air study: see pneumoencephalogram.

alpha rhythm: a descriptive term used in EEG reports for waves which occur 8–11 times per second.

amino acids: a group of related chemical substances found in protein.

amplitude: a term used to describe the height of EEG waves in microvolts.

akinetic seizure: a type of seizure characterized by stiffening of the arms and a sudden falling forward. There are no jerking movements during its brief duration.

angiogram: an x-ray of a blood vessel which has been filled with a radiopaque material.

anticonvulsant: a drug given specifically to reduce the incidence of seizures.

athetoid cerebral palsy: a form of cerebral palsy characterized by slow writhing motions.

aura: a subjective sensation that precedes a grand mal seizure in some individuals.

beta rhythm: a descriptive term used in EEG reports for waves which occur 11–25 times per second.

brain abscess: a localized collection of infected material within the brain substance.

brain-damaged or **brain-injured:** these terms have been used in more than one way.

1). Definite neurological evidence of structural damage, the manifestations of which would be abnormal at any age (as in cerebral palsy); 2). A description of behavior (hyperactive, distractible, impulsive, short attention span) which are thought by the observer to be related to central nervous system damage or dysfunction, with or without definite neurologic findings; 3). Developmental delays (behavior which would be normal for a younger child) which are thought by the observer to be related to brain dysfunction; 4). A description of a group of children whose responses to psychological tests are similar to those of children known to have had significant injury of the central nervous system. These children may or may not have any of the characteristics listed above or have a history of injury.

brain-damaged child: (see cerebral dysfunction)

brain ventricle: one of four normally occurring cavities within the brain.

cerebral dysfunction: a term often used to describe a child who is distractible, clumsy, and hyperactive and who has a short attention span. His ability to reproduce simple geometric figures or other tasks requiring perceptual motor ability is usually poor, but his memory for isolated events is likely to be amazingly good. (see also brain damage)

cerebral palsy: a motor handicap caused by an injury or malformation of the brain.

clonic movement: rhythmic jerking of the body or an extremity.

convulsion (spell, fit, or seizure): a loss or alteration of consciousness accompanied by rhythmic, repetitive jerking.

cryptogenic epilepsy: (see idiopathic epilepsy)

digit-span test: a test wherein an individual is asked to repeat or write a list of numbers after it has been read to him, used to test short-term memory of abstract symbols.

drug idiosyncrasy: an unusual individual reaction to a particular drug.

dyslexia: inability to read at a level expected by age and ability in other areas of development.

Echoencephalogram: a test which records sound waves in a fashion similar to Sonar. A change occurs as the sound waves go through fluids or tissues of different densities.

EEG: (see electroencephalogram)

electroencephalogram: a graphic record of the electrical discharges given off by certain parts of the brain and detected by means of electrodes placed on the scalp.

encephalitis: an inflammation of the brain.

epilepsy: recurrent seizures.

febrile convulsion: a grand mal seizure which occurs in association with a high fever caused by an infection outside the central nervous system.

grand mal seizure: a generalized convulsion characterized by loss of consciousness and stiffening, followed by jerking movements.

Hertz (Hz): the measure of frequency, corresponding to cycles per second.

hypoglycemia: a level of blood sugar (glucose) lower than normal.

hypsarhythmia: a specific electroencephalographic abnormality characterized by a high-voltage 1- to 2-per-second spike-and-wave pattern.

idiopathic: from an unknown cause.

idiopathic epilepsy: recurrent seizures of unknown cause.

IQ (See also intelligence quotient): by definition, a constant value under circumstances of normal mental, physical, and social well-being.

inborn error of metabolism: a hereditary disturbance of the biochemical processes in the body leading to a variety of different symptoms.

infantile myoclonic seizure: (Infantile spasm, lightning major, jackknife epilepsy). A seizure characterized by a sudden dropping of the head and flexion of the arms.

intelligence quotient: the score on a test of intelligence in which the child's performance is compared with other children of his own age. Ordinarily the value is expected to remain reasonably constant for a child (within errors of measurement) over a period of time. Formerly, IQ was defined simply as $MA/CA \times 100$ (mental age divided by chronological age $\times 100$). In recent years it has been more precisely defined for statistical purposes as the degree to which the received score deviates from the average of children his own age.

ketones: a group of chemically related compounds, the end-products of fat breakdown, which can appear in the urine as a result of faulty carbohydrate metabolism.

ketotic hypoglycemia: a condition characterized by low blood sugar and ketones in the urine.

learning disability: see cerebral dysfunction.

mental age (MA): a score obtained by asking an individual to answer test questions of increasing difficulty. Norms for each age have been established by preliminary testing so that an accurate comparison can be made between the individual and the "average" person. The younger the child, the fewer items he is expected to complete.

meningitis: an infection of the membranes covering the brain and spinal cord.

metabolism: the combination of physical and chemical processes involved in the maintenance of life.

migraine: recurrent severe headaches often accompanied in childhood by nausea, vomiting, and abdominal pain and followed by sleep.

minor seizure: a short loss of consciousness, often associated with a sudden movement of the arms and legs.

narcolepsy: recurrent sudden, overwhelming desire to sleep during normal activities.

organic epilepsy: recurrent seizures whose cause is known.

petit mal: a loss of consciousness lasting less than 30 seconds, accompanied by a characteristic electroencephalographic pattern.

phenylketonuria: an inherited disturbance in biochemistry characterized by the body's inability to utilize a certain fraction of protein called phenylalanine.

PKU: (see phenylketonuria)

pneumoencephalogram: an x-ray of the head obtained after air has been substituted for spinal fluid.

psychomotor seizure: a seizure characterized by purposeful but inappropriate motor acts.

reflex seizure: a seizure precipitated by various types of stimulation such as touch, pain, smell, or flashing lights.

reliability: in psychological testing, a measure of the consistency of the test. Three types are available: (a) test-retest (how stable is the measure for two or more separate evaluations with the same test); (b) parallel forms (does the person earn equivalent scores on two comparable forms of the test administered at the same time); and (c) internal-consistency (do two halves of a test concur in the scores earned by a given individual).

rhythm: a term used to describe the number of waves per second.

scan: a test in which the accumulation by a particular organ of small amounts of radioactive particles is recorded. The kind of radioactive material is selected for the specific organ—iodine, for example, is used for the thyroid.

scatter: in testing, an inconsistency of a subject's scores on various parts of the test.

self-induced seizures: a seizure deliberately brought on by a child who has a convulsive tendency.

sickle cell anemia: an inherited blood disorder characterized by abnormally shaped red cells.

spastic quadriplegia: a form of cerebral palsy characterized by muscular stiffness and weakness of all four limbs.

status epilepticus: frequent and closely spaced recurrent grand mal seizures which do not respond to anticonvulsant medication.

steroid hormone: a group of chemically related organic substances originating in certain glands of the body.

spastic diplegia: a form of cerebral palsy characterized by muscular stiffness and weakness in both arms and legs.

spastic hemiplegia: a form of cerebral palsy characterized by muscular stiffness and weakness of an arm and leg on the same side of the body.

symptomatic epilepsy: (see organic epilepsy)

syncope: a fainting spell usually caused by a decrease in the flow of blood to the head.

temporal lobe seizure: a psychomotor seizure.

tetany: increased irritability of the muscles manifested by twitching or seizures. There are several different causes.

tonic movement: a stiffening motion of the body or an extremity.

uremia: the presence of certain abnormal substances in the blood which indicate a serious kidney disorder.

validity: in psychology, the ability of a test to measure the characteristics it was designed to measure; freedom from influence by extraneous factors.

voltage: a term used to describe the intensity of an electrical response. (See also *amplitude*.)

APPENDIX 6
USEFUL REFERENCES

Barrow, Roscoe L. and Faving, Howard D.: *Epilepsy and the Law.* New York, Harper and Row, 1966.

Livingston, Samuel: *Living with Epileptic Seizures.* Springfield, Ill., Charles C Thomas, 1963.

Rodin, Ernst A. *The Prognosis of Patients with Epilepsy.* Springfield, Ill., Charles C Thomas, 1968.

Spock, Benjamin: *Baby and Child Care.* New York, Pocket Books, 1969.

Whipple, Dorothy V. *Dynamics of Development: Euthenic Pediatrics.* New York, McGraw-Hill, 1966.

In addition, the Epilepsy Foundation of America (1828 L Street N.W., Washington, D. C. 20036) distributes a great deal of useful literature in the form of pamphlets.

INDEX

"Abdominal epilepsy," 57
Academy of Certified Social Work-
    ers, 115
Acetone level, 39
Achievement tests, 17
Acute seizures, causes of, 6–7
Adolescence, 94–95
    EEG pattern of, 37
    grand mal seizures of, 46
    idiopathic seizures and, 8
Adrenocorticotropic hormone
    (ACTH), minor motor seiz-
    ures and, 53
Adults, child's relationship to, 93,
    108
Air-study (pneumoencephalo-
    gram), 40–41
Akinetic seizures, 53, 57
Alpha rhythm of EEG, 37
Amino acid disorders, 78–79
Amino acid level, testing of, 40
Amphetamines, children and, 104
Anemia
    loss of consciousness and, 60–
    61
    testing for, 38–39
Anesthesia, after-effects of, 41
Angiography, 41
Atarax (Hydroxyzine HCl), 77
Athetoid cerebral palsy, 71

Baby measles (roseola), 48
Barbiturates, 77
Basal ganglia, 71

Bender Drawings (Visual-Motor
    Gestalt Test), 25–26
Benzedrine, 77
Beta rhythm of EEG, 37
Bicycling, convulsive child and, 88–
    89
Birth, premature, 70, 71
Birth injury
    cerebral palsy and, 70
    seizures and, 7
"Blacking out," 58
"Blacky" test, 27
Blood
    calcium level of, 39–40, 50
    carbon dioxide content of, 58
    effect of drugs on, 63, 67
    phenylalanine level of, 78–
    79
Blood chemical determinations, 39–
    40
Blood clots, brain and, 42
Blood disorders, acute seizures and,
    7
Blood pressure, kidney disease
    and, 80
Blood sugar, low, 7, 39, 50, 79–80,
    106–107
Blood urea nitrogen determination,
    39
Bones, x-rays of, 40
Body weight, drug dosage and, 47,
    65–67
Brain
    blood clot in, 42

Brain (continued)
  congenital abnormality of,
    52–53
  electrical discharges of, 4, 13,
    30–38
Brain damage
  cerebral palsy and, 70–71
  EEG and, 34
  infant seizures and, 50
  minor motor seizures and, 53
  recurrent seizures and, 7, 9
Brain hemorrhage, acute seizures
  and, 7
Brain infection, petit mal seizures
  and, 51
Brain-injured child, 34, 74–75
  causes of, 76
  drugs and, 77
  EEG of, 34, 35
  encephalitis and, 76
  minor motor seizures and, 53
  seizures and, 75–76
  special education of, 76–77,
    113
  testing for, 27–28
  tranquilizers and, 103–104
Brain scan, 41
Brain tumors
  air-study and, 41
  echoencephalogram and, 42
  EEG and, 35
  seizures and, 7
  x-ray and, 40
Brain waves, EEG and, 30–38
Breath-holding, loss of consciousness from, 59–61

Calcium level of blood
  infant seizures and, 50
  testing of, 39–40
Calcium metabolism, abnormal, 7,
  40
Carbamazepine (Tegretol), 68
Carbon dioxide of blood, 58
Central nervous system
  akinetic seizures and, 53
  degenerative disease of, 7, 35,
    77–78

  infection of, 48, 50
  minor motor seizures and, 52
  seizures and, 7–10
Cerebral biopsy, 77–78
Cerebral dysfunction, 34, 74–75
  causes of, 76
  drugs and, 77
  EEG and, 34, 35
  encephalitis and, 76
  seizures and, 53, 75–76
  special education and, 76–77,
    113
  testing for, 27–28
  tranquilizers and, 103–104
Cerebral palsy, 35, 98
  air-study and, 40
  causes and types of, 70–71
Clonic phase of grand mal seizures, 46, 49
College
  stress of, 110
  application for, 111–112
Complete blood count (CBC), 38–
  39
Community services
  convulsive child and, 112–115
  failures of, 116–117
  improvement of, 117–118
Consultant, parents interview with,
  11–16
Conditioning, reflex seizures and,
  53–54
Congenital abnormality of brain,
  52–53
Congenital heart disease, EEG and,
  34
Congenital spastic hemiplegia, 70–
  71
Consciousness
  nonconvulsive loss of, 57–61
  seizures and alteration of, 4–5
Contact sports, convulsive child
  and, 89
Control of seizures, 62–63, 69–70
Copper metabolism disorder, 79
Coproporphyrin, 39
Cortisone, hypoglycemia and, 79
Coughing tic, 62

Counseling services for parents, 114–115
Cryptogenic seizures, 6
Curriculum of school, 102

Day care centers, 105–106, 113
Dé jà vu, 5
Denver Developmental Screening Test (DDST), 21, 23–24
Developmental stages of childhood, 14–15
Dexidrine, 77
Diabetes
    EEG and, 34
    low blood sugar and, 80
Diagnosis of seizures, 8–11
    chemical and surgical tests for, 38–42
    consultant's role in, 11–12
    EEG and, 30–38
    medical history and, 12–13
    neurological examination for, 15–16
    psychological testing and, 16–30
Diagnostic center of community, 113
Diet
    ketogenic, 68–69
    low phenylalanine, 79
Dilantin (diphenyhydantoin)
    effects and use of, 66–67
    high blood pressure and, 80
    liquid form of, 64, 66
    petit mal seizures and, 52
    treatment of grand mal seizures and, 47
Dilantin level, testing of, 40
Diphenylhydantoin, see Dilantin
Dostoevski, Fyodor, 5
Draw-A-Man test, 26
Driving, convulsive child and, 96–97
Drugs, 62
    administration of, 63–64
    adolescent and, 95–96
    cerebral dysfunction and, 77
    dosage of, 47, 65–67

effect on blood by, 63, 67
effect on EEG by, 35
types of, 64–68
See also Medication

Ear infections, febrile seizures and, 48
Echoencephalogram, 42
Education
    cerebral dysfunction and, 76–77, 113
    convulsive child and, 97–107, 113
    learning disability and, 76–77, 113
    mental retardation and, 71, 73–74, 97–99, 104–106, 113
    Montessori method of, 100–101
    necessity of, 107
    remedial, 113
    See also Schools
EEG, *see* Electroencephalograph
Electrical discharges of brain
    seizures and, 4, 13
    EEG and, 30–38
Electroencephalograph (EEG), 4, 9, 13, 67
    abnormal findings of, 35–38, 55–56
    of adolescents, 37
    akinetic seizures and, 53
    brain damage and, 34
    childhood migraines and, 57
    description of, 30
    effect of drugs on, 35
    febrile seizures and, 49
    findings of, 31–32
    grand mal seizures and, 38, 47
    minor motor seizures and, 53
    of newborn infant, 37, 50
    petit mal seizures and, 38, 51
    preparation of child for, 31
    psychomotor seizures and, 52
    unconsciousness and, 61
    uses of, 33–35
Employment
    application for, 110–111

Employment (*continued*)
  choice of, 108–110
  counseling for, 114
Encephalitis, 6, 9, 49
  cerebral dysfunction and, 76
  minor motor seizures and, 52–53
Environmental seizures (reflex), 43–54
Epilepsia seizure, 6
Epilepsy
  "abdominal," 57
  definition of, 6
  driver's license laws and, 96–97
  employment and, 110–111
  marriage laws and, 112
  misconceptions of, 90
Experience of seizures, 5–6
Eyeblinking tic, 62

Facial twitching tic, 62
Fainting, 58
Fasting blood sugar test, 39
Febrile seizures, 4, 10, 71
  causes and treatment of, 47, 48–49
  phenobarbital and, 65
Fever
  acute seizures and, 6
  febrile seizures and, 48–49
  grand mal seizures and, 47
  treatment of, 49
First aid, grand mal seizures and, 46
Football, convulsive child and, 89
Form of EEG, 35–37
Frequency of EEG, 35

Gas chromatography, 66
"Gilles de la Tourette" tic, 62
Glucagon, 80
Grand mal seizures, 59, 98
  description of, 45–46
  Dilantin and, 47, 66
  EEG of, 33–34, 38, 47
  first aid for, 46
  petit mal seizures and, 51

Mysoline for, 68
Tegretol and, 68
treatment of, 47–48, 52
Tridione and, 67
Gums, swelling of, 66

Habit spasm, 61–62
Hallucinations, marihuana and, 96
Haloperidol, 62
Handicapped children
  care of, 105–107, 113
  education of, 97–99
Headaches, *see* Migraine
Heart disease, congenital, 34, 58
Hemophilia, acute seizures and, 7
Heredity of seizures, 112
Heroin, infant withdrawal from, 50
Hertz waves of EEG, 37
Horseback riding, convulsive child and, 89
Hyperkinetic child, 75
Hyperplasia of gums, 66
Hypoglycemia, causes and treatment of, 79–80, 106–107
Hypsarhythmia, 38, 53
Hysteria, 59

Ice skating, convulsive child and, 90
Idiopathic mental retardation, 40
Idiopathic seizures, 4, 6–8, 10, 69
  air-study and, 40
  grand mal, 46, 48
  self-induced seizures and, 54
Idiosyncrasy to drugs, 63
Illinois Test of Psycholinguistic Abilities (ITPA), 27–28
Independence, child's development of, 11, 91–92, 107–108
Infantile myoclonic seizures (minor motor seizures), 4, 16
  central nervous system and, 52
  EEG of, 38
  PKU and, 79
  treatment of, 53
  Valium and, 68

Infants
    causes of seizures in, 7–8
    developmental stages of, 14–15
    EEG of, 37
    neurological examination of, 15–16
    PKU testing of, 79
    "seal bark" of, 61
    seizures of, 49–50
Infections
    cerebral dysfunction and, 76
    febrile seizures and, 48
    nervous system, 48, 50
    seizures and, 6–7
Intelligence
    definition of, 19
    measurement of, 17–19
Intelligence quotient (IQ), 17, 24, 25
    definition of, 19–20
    mental retardation and, 73–74
    special education and, 105
IQ, see Intelligence quotient
Iron deficiency anemia, 60–61

Jamais vu, 5

Ketogenic diet, 68–69
Ketosis, 68–69
Ketotic hypoglycemia
    testing for, 39
    treatment of, 80
Kidneys, Triodione and, 67
Kidney disease
    seizures and, 7, 80
    test for, 39
Kindergarten, 99–100

Lead poisoning
    cerebral dysfunction and, 76
    seizures and, 9, 80–81
    testing for, 39, 40
Learning disability, 74–75
    causes of, 76
    drugs and, 77
    EEG and, 34, 35
    minor motor seizures and, 53

special education and, 76–77, 113
    testing for, 27–28
    tranquilizers and, 103–104
Leucine, 79
Light-induced seizures, 54–55
    driving and, 96
Lightning major attacks, 4
Little's disease, 71
Low blood sugar
    causes and treatment of, 79–80, 106–107
    infant seizures and, 50
    recurrent convulsions and, 7
    testing for, 39
Low blood calcium
    infant seizures and, 50
    testing for, 39–40

Maple Syrup Urine Disease, 79
Marihuana, seizures and, 95–96
Marriage laws, epilepsy and, 112
Maturity rates, 101
Mebaral (mephobarbital)
    psychomotor seizures and, 52
    use of, 67
Medical history
    diagnosis and, 12–13
    job applications and, 110–111
Medication
    administering to children, 62–63
    adolescents and, 95–96
    for akinetic seizures, 53
    body weight and dosage of, 47, 65–67
    childhood illness and, 100
    febrile seizures and, 49
    for grand mal seizures, 47–48, 66–68
    for minor motor seizures, 53
    petit mal seizures and, 51
    psychomotor seizures and, 52
    reflex seizures and, 53, 54
    school and, 102–104
    See also Drugs
Medium-chain triglycerides (MCT), 69

Meningitis, 6, 48, 71
Mental age
    IQ test and, 20
    testing for, 26
Mental retardation
    air-study and, 40
    education and, 71, 73–74, 97–
        99, 104–106, 113
    EEG and, 35
    IQ and, 73
    nursery school and, 99
    petit mal seizures and, 51
    PKU and, 79
    seizures and, 10, 17, 71–73
Mephobarbital (Mebaral), psycho-
    motor seizures, and, 52,
    67
Metabolism disorders, 78–79
Migraine, childhood, 55–57, 58
Minor motor seizures (infantile
    myoclonic seizures), 4, 16
    central nervous system and,
        52
    EEG of, 38
    PKU and, 79
    treatment of, 53
    Valium and, 68
Misconceptions of seizures, 10–11,
    85–86, 91, 98
Montessori, Maria, 100
Montessori method, 100–101
Motor skills, testing of, 23–25
Myoclonic seizures, see Infantile
    myoclonic seizures
Mysoline (primidone)
    akinetic seizures and, 53
    effects of, 68
    psychomotor seizures and, 52

Narcolepsy, 57, 58
Nervous system, see Central nerv-
    ous system
Neurological examination of child,
    12, 15–16
Nodding spasms, 61
Nonrecurrent seizures, causes of,
    6–7
Normalcy, standard of, 72

Nursery school, 99, 115
Nurses, public health, 114

Oxygen loss
    blackouts from, 59–61
    seizures and, 7
Organic epilepsy, 6

Parents
    adolescent and, 94–95
    anxiety of, 12–13
    attitudes toward convulsive
        child, 8–11, 86–88
    child's independence and, 91–
        92
    counseling for, 114–115
    explanation to child, 90–91
    psychological testing and, 16–
        19
Peabody Picture Vocabulary Test,
    21, 23
Peer relationships of child, 92–93,
    108
Personality, testing of, 26–27
Petit mal seizures, 4, 10, 16
    EEG of, 38, 51
    heredity of, 112
    medication for, 67–68
    PKU and, 79
    self-induced, 54, 55
    symptoms of, 50–51
    treatment for, 51–52
Phenobarbital, 67
    dosage of, 65–66
    effects of, 64–65
    elixir of, 63
    febrile seizures and, 49
    grand mal seizures and, 47
    high blood pressure and, 80
    for migraines, 57
    petit mal seizures and, 51, 52,
        68
    reflex seizures and, 54
Phenobarbital level test, 40
Phenylalanine level of blood, 78–79
Phenylketonuria (PKU), 78–79
    EEG and, 35
    idiopathic seizures and, 7
    testing for, 39, 40, 79

Phenylpyruvic acid, 39
Physician, parents' relationship to, 8–9, 86–87
PKU, see Phenylketonuria
Pneumoencephalogram (air-study), 40–41
Poisoning
    cerebral dysfunction and, 76
    by lead, 9, 39, 40, 80–81
    seizures and, 7
Poliomyelitis, 70
Premature births, cerebral palsy and, 70–71
Psychological tests
    IQ and, 19–20
    limitations of, 20–21, 25, 26, 27
    purpose of, 16–19
    report from, 28, 30
    screening tests for, 17, 21–24
    specialized types of, 24–28
Psychomotor seizures, 4, 5, 51
    Mebaral and, 52
    Mysoline and, 68
Public health nurses, 114
Public health services
    inadequacy of, 116–117
    improvement of, 117–118
Pyridoxine (vitamin B₆), deficiency of, 50

Recurrent seizures, 6
    causes of, 7–8
    driver's licenses and, 96–97
Reflex seizures (environmental), 53–54
Residential centers, 106–107, 114
"Retarded educable" child, schooling of, 104–105
"Retarded trainable" child, 71, 74
Rickets, 40
Ritalin (methylphenidate), 77
Rorschach (Ink-Blot) Test, 27
Roseola (baby measles), 48

School
    attitudes of, 8, 97, 102–103
    choice of, 98–99, 101–102

retarded classes in, 104–105
    tranquilizers and, 103–104
School psychology tests, 17–18
"Screening" tests, 17, 21–24
"Seal bark," infants and, 61
Sedatives, 77
    EEG readings and, 35
    phenobarbital as, 64–65
Self-induced seizures, 54–55
Sickle cell anemia, testing for, 39
Sickle cell disease, acute seizures and, 7
Side-effects of drugs, 63
Skiing, convulsive child and, 90
Sniffling tic, 62
Social workers, role of, 115–116
Spastic diplegia, 71
Spastic quadriplegia, 71
Sports, child's participation in, 88–90
Stanford-Binet Test, 25
Status epilepticus, 46
    drug stoppage and, 65
    Valium and, 68
Steroid drugs, 35
Swimming
    convulsive child and, 89
    oxygen depletion during, 58–59
Symptomatic epilepsy, 6
Syphilis, seizures and, 7

Tay-Sachs disease, 77
Teachers
    attitudes of toward child, 97–99, 102–103
    of retarded children, 104
Tegretol (carbamazepine), 68
Temporal lobe seizures, 5
Tetany, seizures and, 7, 80
Thematic Apperception Test (TAT), 26–27
Thorazine (chlorpromazine), 77
Throat infections, febrile seizures and, 48
Thyroid extract drugs, 35
Thyroid problems, EEG and, 34
Tic spasms, 61–62

Tonic phase of grand mal seizure, 46, 49

Tranquilizers, learning disabilities and, 103–104

Tridione (trimethidione), use and effect of, 67

Urinalysis, 39

Valium (diazepam), anticonvulsant use of, 68

Verbal skills, testing of, 24–25

Vineland Social Maturity Scale, 21–23

Vistaril (hydroxyzine pamoate), 77

Vitamin B₆ (pyridoxine), deficiency of, 50

Vocabulary, testing of, 23

Vocational counseling services, 114

Vocational planning, 108–110

Voltage of EEG, 35

Wechsler Intelligence Scale for Children (WISC), 34–35

Wide Range Achievement Test, 25

Wilson's Disorder, 79

Wisconsin, driver license laws of, 97

X-rays, diagnostic use of, 40

Zarontin (ethosuximide) petit mal seizures and, 51, 67 uses and effects of, 67–68